THE SPORTS REHABILITATION THERAPISTS' GUIDEBOOK

The Sports Rehabilitation Therapists' Guidebook is a well-equipped, comprehensive, practical, evidence-based guide that seeks to assist both students and graduate sport practitioners. The book is designed to be a quick-reference book during assessment and treatment planning, giving instant access to figures and case scenarios. It introduces evidence-based practice in all principal areas of sport rehabilitation such as anatomy, musculoskeletal assessment, pitch-side care, injury treatment modalities and exercise rehabilitation principles and related areas, and is designed to be more flexible than the usual single-focus books. It is written by a team of expert contributors offering a systematic perspective on core concepts.

The book can be used as a guide in each stage of the sport rehabilitation process and it is an asset for sport clinical practitioners such as sport rehabilitators, sport therapists, personal trainers, strength and conditioning coaches, as well as for students on these and related courses in their daily practice on core clinical placements such as a clinic/sporting environment, pitch side and university.

Konstantinos Papadopoulos is Director of Programmes for the postgraduate programmes and Programme Leader for the MSc Sport Rehabilitation at the London Sports Institute, Middlesex University, London.

Mark Richardson is Programme Leader for the BSc Sport and Exercise Rehabilitation and Senior Lecturer at the London Sports Institute, Middlesex University, London.

THE SPORTS REHABILITATION THERAPISTS' GUIDEBOOK

Accessing Evidence-Based Practice

Edited by Konstantinos Papadopoulos and Mark Richardson

Routledge
Taylor & Francis Group

NEW YORK AND LONDON

First published 2022
by Routledge
605 Third Avenue, New York, NY 10158

and by Routledge
2 Park Square, Milton Park, Abingdon, Oxon OX14 4RN

Routledge is an imprint of the Taylor & Francis Group, an informa business

Library of Congress Cataloging-in-Publication Data
Names: Papadopoulos, Konstantinos (Physiotherapist), editor.
Title: The sports rehabilitation therapists' guidebook: accessing evidence-based practice/edited by Konstantinos Papadopoulos and Mark Richardson.
Description: New York, NY: Routledge, 2020. |
Includes bibliographical references and index. |
Identifiers: LCCN 2020055359 (print) | LCCN 2020055360 (ebook) |
ISBN 9780367773892 (hardback) | ISBN 9780367773908 (paperback) |
ISBN 9781003171140 (ebook)
Subjects: LCSH: Sports injuries–Patients–Rehabilitation. |
Sports injuries–Treatment.
Classification: LCC RD97 .S787 2020 (print) |
LCC RD97 (ebook) | DDC 617.1/027–dc23
LC record available at https://lccn.loc.gov/2020055359
LC ebook record available at https://lccn.loc.gov/2020055360

ISBN: 978-0-367-77389-2 (hbk)
ISBN: 978-0-367-77390-8 (pbk)
ISBN: 978-1-003-17114-0 (ebk)

Typeset in Bembo
by Newgen Publishing UK

CONTENTS

FIGURES

TABLES

CONTRIBUTORS

Konstantinos Papadopoulos, PhD, is Director of Programmes for the LSI postgraduate programmes in the Faculty of Science and Technology at Middlesex University, London. As a senior lecturer, he has been leading the MSc Sport Rehabilitation programme for the last four years. He is a Health & Care Professional Council registered physiotherapist with a research focus on sports injuries. Konstantinos was a National Health Service honorary researcher for five years and has published a number of research papers in peer-reviewed journals. He holds an MSc in Exercise Rehabilitation, a PhD in Healthcare Sciences and he is also a Senior Fellow in the Higher Education Academy.

Mark Richardson achieved BSc Honours in Exercise and Health Science before going on to study Physiotherapy followed by an MSc in Sport and Exercise Rehabilitation. As a Chartered Physiotherapist, Mark has worked for the National Health Service, the Ministry of Defence, the private sector as well as for various sport teams, such as England Touch Rugby and GB Canoeing. Mark is currently Senior Lecturer, Higher Education Academy Fellow and Programme Leader for the Sport & Exercise Rehabilitation degree programme at Middlesex University, London.

Ebony Fewkes completed her MSc in Sports Rehabilitation. As a British Association of Sport Rehabilitators and Trainers (BASRaT) accredited Sports Rehabilitator she currently works with Saracens RFU, within the women's team, and has previously worked in Australian Rules Football. Ebony is currently a lecturer, Higher Education Academy Fellow and Programme Leader for the Sport & Exercise Rehabilitation degree programme at Middlesex University, London.

Alex Anzelmo's first degree was a BSc in Sports Science at Manchester Metropolitan University (MMU). After a stint in Italy playing professional basketball he returned to the UK and undertook a PGCE/in secondary education (Brunel), followed by a BSc in Physiotherapy (Brunel), MSc in Sports Injuries and Rehabilitation (MMU) and read for a PhD at Hertfordshire University. He was on the GB Olympic medical team for 11 years and the Olympic physio committee for the same period. During this time, he worked with several teams/sports at various training camps, World, European, Commonwealth and Olympic Games. He was head physio and senior governing body physio for GB & NI Basketball from 1996 to 2004 inclusive.

Mark Adamoulas has worked in an applied capacity for over ten years in both sport and business environments. Having started his journey on a generic sport degree, he was fascinated by the mental side of athletic performance, and subsequently pursued an MSc in Applied Sport and Exercise Psychology. His doctoral research is around the key psychological qualities athletes on talent pathways must possess in order to reach the elite level. He has held lecturing posts at four UK universities, the most recent in 2017. Outside academia, he has worked with English Premier League football, Formula 1, numerous individual athletes, and as an executive coach within a number of FTSE 100 companies.

Sarah Budd holds a BSc in Sports Rehabilitation and an MSc in Sports Massage, Therapy and Rehabilitation. She is a British Association of Sport Rehabilitators and Trainers (BASRaT) accredited Sports Rehabilitator and she currently works with Tottenham Hotspur women's team. She is a Higher Education Academy Fellow.

PREFACE

The Sports Rehabilitation Therapists' Guidebook is a well-equipped, comprehensive, practical, evidence-based guide (pocketbook) to assist both students and graduate sport practitioners. The book is designed to be a memo book during assessment and treatment planning with instant access to figures and case scenarios.

It introduces evidence-based practice in all principal areas of sport rehabilitation such as anatomy, musculoskeletal assessment, pitch-side care, injury treatment modalities and exercise rehabilitation principles and is not the typical inflexible textbook designed for one module only.

It can be used as a guide in each stage of the sport rehabilitation process and it is an asset for sport clinical practitioners such as sport rehabbers, sport therapists, personal trainers, strength and conditioning coaches and students in their daily practice on core clinical placements such as a clinic/sporting environment, pitch side and university.

It is written by a team of expert contributors offering a systematic perspective on core concepts. All authors are academics (sport physiotherapists, sport rehabilitators or psychologists) who teach in higher education institutions.

The book is divided into seven main chapters. The first two chapters present in detail the anatomy of the musculoskeletal system and how muscles and the most common conditions can be assessed. Chapter 3 reports the most common sport injuries of the joints along with the mechanism of injury, symptoms and the most updated evidence-based treatment. Chapter 4 presents the pitch-side care and player management such as taping, first aid and concussion assessment and management. Chapter 5 presents the most common injury treatment modalities used by the sport therapist/rehabilitator. Chapter 6 includes the principles of exercise and rehabilitation, and the last chapter presents the academic and research method skills that the sport practitioner needs to master.

1

NEURO-MUSCULOSKELETAL ANATOMY

Mark Richardson

Bones

The human skeleton is the internal framework of the human body (Figure 1.1, 1.2), it is divided into the axial skeleton which is formed by the vertebral column, the rib cage, the skull and other associated bones and the appendicular skeleton which is attached to the axial skeleton and is formed by the shoulder girdle, the pelvic girdle and the bones of the upper limb and lower limb. The human skeleton performs six functions support, movement, protection, production of blood cells, storage of minerals, and endocrine regulation [5].

Human Skeleton System Anatomy

Cranium

Maxilla

Mandible

Cervical Vertebrae
C1 - C7

Clavicle

Manubrium

Scapula

Scapula

Sternum

Ribs

Humerus

Humerus

Lumbar Vertebrae
L1 - L5

Radius

Ulna

Pelvis

Sacral Vertebrae
S1 - S5

Carpals

Metacarpals

Pubis

Phalanges

Femur

Femur

Patella

Patella

Fibula

Fibula

Tibia

Tibia

Tarsals

Metatarsals

Phalanges

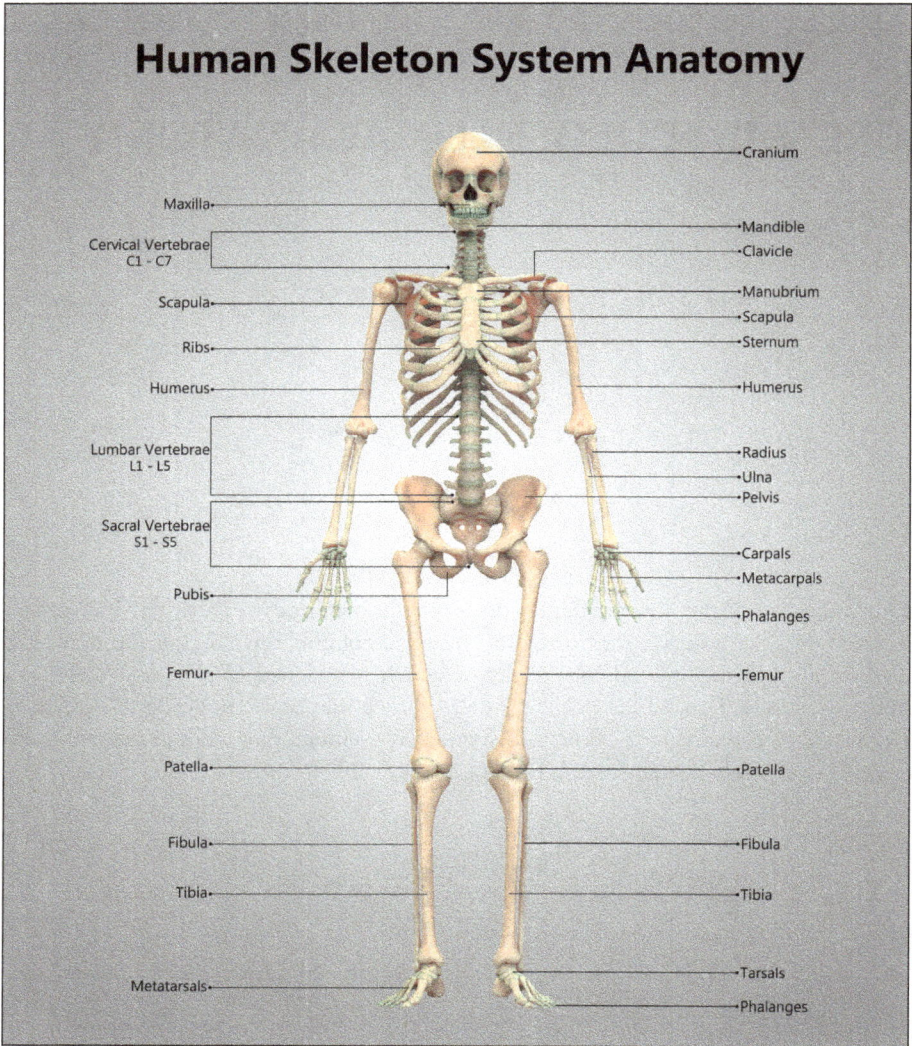

FIGURE 1.1 Anterior view of the human skeleton anatomy.

Human Skeleton System Anatomy

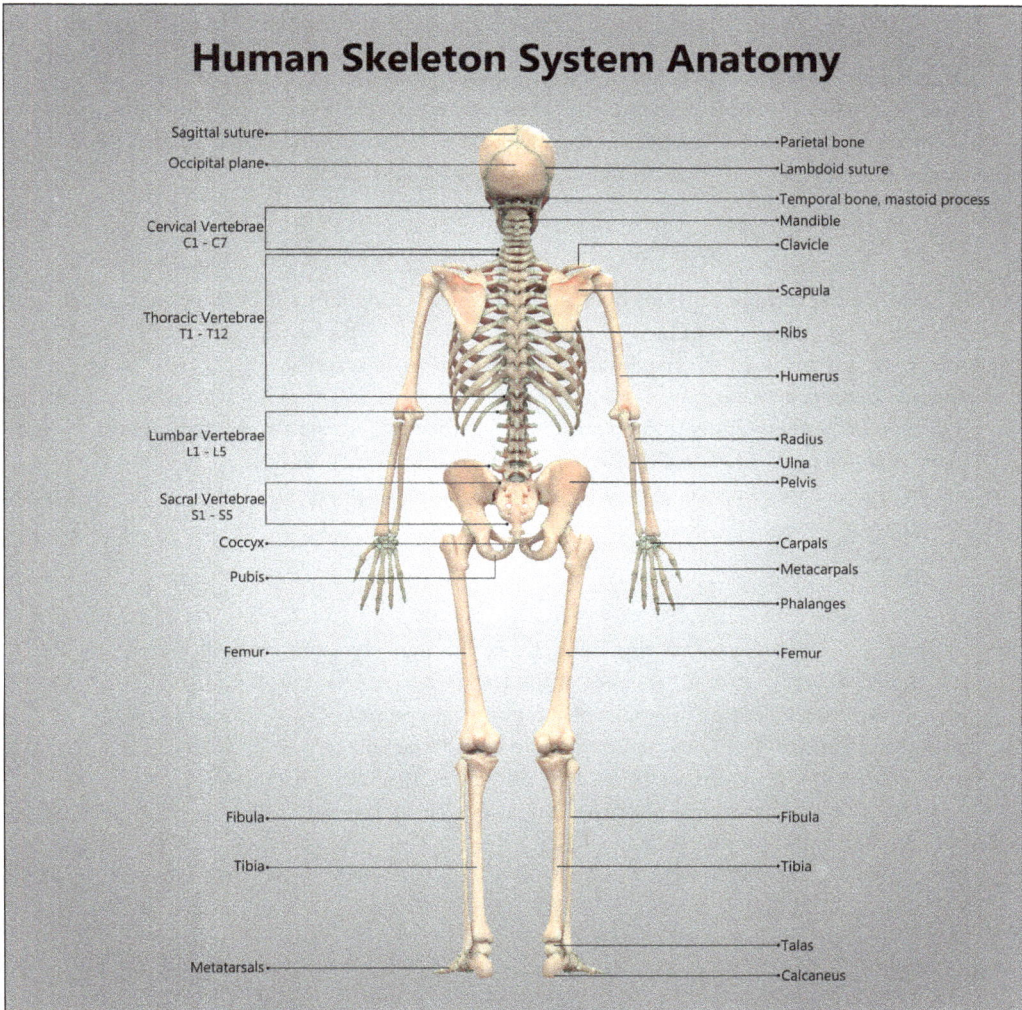

Sagittal suture
Occipital plane
Cervical Vertebrae C1 - C7
Thoracic Vertebrae T1 - T12
Lumbar Vertebrae L1 - L5
Sacral Vertebrae S1 - S5
Coccyx
Pubis
Femur
Fibula
Tibia
Metatarsals

Parietal bone
Lambdoid suture
Temporal bone, mastoid process
Mandible
Clavicle
Scapula
Ribs
Humerus
Radius
Ulna
Pelvis
Carpals
Metacarpals
Phalanges
Femur
Fibula
Tibia
Talas
Calcaneus

FIGURE 1.2 Posterior view of the human skeleton anatomy.

Muscles

Head and Neck

Sternocleidomastoid

Origin: Anterior and superior manubrium and superior medial third of clavicle.

Insertion: Lateral aspect of mastoid process and anterior half of superior nuchal line of occipital bone.

Action: Flexes and laterally rotates cervical spine. Protracts head when acting together. Extends neck when neck already partially extended.

Nerve: Spinal accessory nerve (XI) (lateral roots C1–5).

Levator Scapulae

Origin: Posterior tubercle of transverse processes of C1–4.
Insertion: Medial border of scapula between superior angle and base of spine of scapula.
Action: Elevates, medially rotates and retracts scapula, extends and laterally flexes neck.
Nerve: Cervical nerve (C3–C4) and dorsal scapular nerve (C5).

Trapezius

Origin: Medial third of superior nuchal line; external occipital protuberance, nuchal ligament and spinous processes of C7–T12 vertebrae.
Insertion: Lateral third of clavicle, acromion and spine of scapula.
Action: *Upper fibres* elevate pectoral girdle and scapula. *Middle fibres* retract scapula. *Lower fibres* depress shoulders. Upper and lower fibres together rotate scapula upwards. *Bilateral contraction* extends neck. *Unilateral contraction* ipsilateral side flexion of neck.
Nerve: Accessory nerve (CN XI – motor). Cervical nerves (C3 and C4 – pain and proprioception).

Scalenes

Origin: *Scalenus Anterior*: Anterior tubercles of the transverse processes of vertebrae C3–C6.
  Scalenus Medius: Posterior tubercles of the transverse processes of vertebrae C2–C7.
Scalenus Posterior: Posterior tubercles of the transverse processes of vertebrae C5–C7.
Insertion: *Scalenus Anterior*: Scalene tubercle of the first rib.
Scalenus Medius: Upper surface of the first rib behind the subclavian artery.
Scalenus Posterior: Lateral surface of the second rib.
Action: Flexes and rotates neck.
Nerve: *Scalenus Anterior*: Brachial plexus, C5–C7. *Scalenus Medius*: Brachial plexus, C3–C8.

Scalenus Posterior: Brachial plexus, C7–C8.
Splenius Capitis

Origin: Lower half of ligamentum nuchae (C4–C6) and spinous process of C7–T3.
Insertion: Superior nuchal line. Mastoid process of temporal bone and rough surface adjoining occipital bone.
Action: *Acting bilaterally* extension of the head and cervical spine. *Acting unilaterally* lateral flexion of the head and neck and rotation the head to the same side.

Splenius Cervicis

Origin: Spinous processes of T3 to T6.
Insertion: Posterior tubercles of transverse processes of C1 to C3.
Action: *Bilaterally* they extend the neck. *Unilaterally* they laterally flex and rotate the head and neck to the contralateral side.
Nerve: Dorsal rami of cervical spinal nerves (C5–C8).

Rectus Capitis Anterior

Origin: Anterior surface of the lateral mass of the atlas (C1 vertebra) and the root of its transverse process.
Insertion: The inferior surface of the occipital bone anterior to the foramen magnum.
Action: Aids in flexion of the head and the neck.
Nerve: C1, C2.

Rectus Capitis Lateralis

Origin: Superior surfaces of the transverse processes of the atlas.
Insertion: Inferior surface of the jugular process of the occipital bone.
Action: Stabilises the head and weakly assists with lateral flexion of the head.
Nerve: Anterior primary rami of the first cervical spinal nerve (C1).

Rectus Capitis Posterior Minor

Origin: Tubercle on the posterior arch of the atlas (C1).
Insertion: Medial portion of the inferior nuchal line of the occipital bone.
Action: Extension of the head.
Nerve: Suboccipital nerve or dorsal ramus of cervical spinal nerve (C1).

Rectus Capitis Posterior Major

Origin: Tip of the spinous process of the axis (C2).
Insertion: Lateral aspect of the inferior nuchal line of the occiput, also the bone inferior to this line.
Action: Extends and rotates atlanto-occipital joint.
Nerve: Suboccipital nerve or dorsal ramus of cervical spinal nerve (C1).

Longus Capitis

Origin: Anterior tubercles of transverse processes of C3–C6 vertebrae.
Insertion: Inferior surfaces of the basilar portion of the occipital bone.
Action: *Acting bilaterally* flexion of the cervical vertebrae and head. *Acting unilaterally* rotation and lateral flexion of the cervical vertebrae and head to the contralateral side.
Nerve: Muscular branches of C1 – C4.

Longissimus Capitis

Origin: Posterior surface of transverse processes of T1–T5 and the articular tubercle of C4–C7.
Insertion: Posterior margin of mastoid process and the temporal bone.
Action: *Acting bilaterally*, extends and hyperextends head. *Acting unilaterally*, flexes and rotates the head ipsilaterally.
Nerve: Dorsal rami of cervical and thoracic spinal nerves (C6 to T4).

Longus Colli

> **Origin**: Anterior tubercles and anterior surfaces of bodies of C3–T3. Superior oblique portion arises from anterior tubercles of the transverse processes of the C3, C4, C5. Inferior oblique portion arises from the front of the bodies of T1, T2, T3. Vertical portion arises from the front of the bodies of T1, T2, T3 and C5, C6, C7.
>
> **Insertion**: Anterior arch of atlas, anterior tubercles of C5–6, anterior surfaces of bodies of vertebrae C2–4. Superior oblique portion inserts into the tubercle on the anterior arch of the atlas. Inferior oblique portion into the anterior tubercles of the transverse processes of C5, C6. Vertical portion into the front of the bodies of the C2, C3, C4.
>
> **Action**: Cervical flexion, ipsilateral side flexion and some cervical rotation.
>
> **Nerve**: C2–6 Ventral rami.

Trunk

Rectus Abdominus

> **Origin**: Pubic symphysis, pubic crest.
>
> **Insertion**: Xiphoid process, Costal cartilages of ribs 5–7.
>
> **Action**: Trunk flexion, expiration.
>
> **Nerve**: Intercostal nerves (T6–T11), Subcostal nerve (T12).

Internal Obliques

> **Origin**: Anterior two-thirds of iliac crest, iliopectineal arch, thoracolumbar fascia.
>
> **Insertion**: Inferior borders of ribs 10–12, linea alba, pubic crest and pectin pubis (via conjoint tendon).
>
> **Action**: *Bilateral contraction* trunk flexion, compresses abdominal viscera, expiration. *Unilateral contraction* trunk lateral flexion (ipsilateral), trunk rotation (ipsilateral).
>
> **Nerve**: Intercostal nerves (T7–T11), subcostal nerve (T12), iliohypogastric nerve (L1), ilioinguinal nerve (L1).

External Obliques

> **Origin**: External surfaces of ribs 5–12.
>
> **Insertion**: Linea alba, pubic tubercle, anterior half of iliac crest.
>
> **Action**: *Bilateral contraction* trunk flexion, compresses abdominal viscera, expiration. *Unilateral contraction* trunk lateral flexion (ipsilateral), trunk rotation (contralateral).
>
> **Nerve**: Intercostal nerves (T7–T11), Subcostal nerve (T12), Iliohypogastric nerve (L1).

Quadratus Lumborum

> **Origin**: Iliolumbar ligament and internal lip of posterior iliac crest.
>
> **Insertion**: Medial half of lower border of 12th rib and tips of transverse processes of lumbar vertebrae.
>
> **Action**: Lateral flexes the vertebral column. Extends lumbar vertebrae.
>
> **Nerve**: Subcostal nerve (T12). Iliohypogastric and ilioinguinal nerve (both from L1). Branches from the ventral rami (L2 and L3).

Erector Spinae (Iliocostalis, Longissimus, Spinalis)
Illiocostalis

> **Origin**: Anterior surface of a broad and thick tendon attached to the medial crest of the sacrum, spinous processes of the lumbar vertebrae, T11 and T12. Posterior part of the medial lip of iliac crest, supra-spinous ligament and the lateral crest of sacrum.
> **Insertion**: By tendons into inferior borders of the angles of the lower 6 or 7 ribs.
> **Action**: *Unilaterally*, laterally flexes the spine. *Bilaterally*, extension and hyperextension of the spine. Respiration, it assists as an accessory muscle of expiration.
> **Nerve**: Dorsal rami of thoracic and lumbar spinal nerves (T7 to L3).

Longissimus

> **Origin**: Transverse and spinous processes of lumbar vertebrae and thoracolumbar fascia.
> **Insertion**: Transverse process of all thoracic vertebrae and the lower 9 or 10 ribs between the tubercles and angles.
> **Action**: *Unilaterally*, extension of vertebral column and flexion to the contralateral side. *Bilaterally*, extension and hyperextension of vertebral column.
> **Nerve**: Dorsal rami of thoracic and lumbar spinal nerves (T7 to L5).

Spinalis

> **Origin**: Lower part of ligamentum nuchae (C4 to C6) and spinous process of C7–T2.
> **Insertion**: Spinous processes of C2 and the 3rd and 4th cervical spinous process.
> **Action**: *Bilaterally*, extend the spine. *Unilaterally*, laterally flex and rotate the spine contralateral side.
> **Nerve**: Dorsal rami of cervical and thoracic spinal nerves (C4 to T1).

Semispinalis Capitis

> **Origin**: Articular processes of C5–7 and transverse processes of T1–T6.
> **Insertion**: Occiput in between the superior and inferior nuchal line.
> **Action**: *Bilaterally* extension of the head and neck. *Unilaterally* rotation of head and neck to (ipsilateral).
> **Nerve**: Greater occipital nerve.

Semispinalis Cervicis

> **Origin**: Transverse processes of T1 to T6, articular processes of C4–C7.
> **Insertion**: Spinous processes of C2 to C5.
> **Action**: *Bilaterally*: extension of the cervical spine. *Unilaterally*: lateral flexion of the neck and rotation (ipsilateral).
> **Nerve**: Dorsal rami of cervical spinal nerves.

Semispinalis Thoracis

> **Origin**: Transverse processes of vertebrae T6–T10.
> **Insertion**: Spinous processes of vertebrae C6–T4.

Action: *Bilaterally*: extension of head, cervical and thoracic spine. *Unilaterally*: lateral flexion of head, cervical and thoracic spine (ipsilateral), rotation of head, cervical and thoracic spine (contralateral).

Nerve: Medial branches of posterior rami of spinal nerves.

Intertransversarii

Origin: Lateral lumbar intertransversarii: transverse and accessory processes of vertebrae L1–L4. Medial lumbar intertransversarii: accessory processes of vertebrae L1–L4.

Insertion: Lateral lumbar intertransversarii: transverse process of succeeding vertebra. Medial lumbar intertransversarii: mammillary processes of succeeding vertebra.

Action: Assists lateral flexion of the spine; stabilises spine.

Nerve: Anterior rami of spinal nerves.

Rotators

Origin: Posterior surface of the superior margin of the transverse process of the thoracic vertebrae.

Insertion: Inferior margin of the lateral aspect of the laminae of the thoracic vertebrae.

Action: *Bilaterally*: extension of thoracic spine. *Unilaterally*: rotation of thoracic spine (contralateral).

Nerve: Medial branches of posterior rami of spinal nerves.

Shoulder Complex

Rhomboid Major

Origin: Spinous processes T2–T5.

Insertion: Medial border of scapula from level of spine to inferior angle.

Action: Retracts the scapula and rotates it to depress the glenoid cavity. Fixes the scapula to the thoracic wall.

Nerve: Dorsal scapular nerve (C4–5).

Rhomboid Minor

Origin: Nuchal ligament, spinous processes C7–T1.

Insertion: Triangular area, medial end of scapular spine.

Action: Scapular retraction, scapular elevation, scapular rotation inferiorly to depress glenoid cavity. Assist serratus anterior to fix scapula to thoracic wall and fix scapula during movements of the upper limb.

Nerve: Dorsal scapular nerve (C5).

Trapezius – See Head and Neck.
Levator Scapulae – See Head and Neck.

Serratus Anterior

Origin: Superior surface of the 8 or 9 upper ribs and intervening intercostal fascia.
Insertion: Anterior border of scapula.
Action: Protraction and lateral rotation of scapula.
Nerve: Long thoracic nerve (C5–7).

Pectoralis Major

Origin: Clavicular head originates from the anterior surface of the medial clavicle. Sternocostal head originates from the anterior surface of the sternum, the superior six costal cartilages and the aponeurosis of the external oblique muscle.
Insertion: Lateral lip of the bicipital groove of the humerus. Crest of the greater tubercle of the humerus.
Action: Adducts, medially rotates, flexes and extends the shoulder.
Nerve: Lateral and medial pectoral nerve, C5–T1.

Pectoralis Minor

Origin: Anterior surfaces of the sternal ends of ribs 3–5.
Insertion: Medial border and upper surface of coracoid process.
Action: Stabilisation, depression, protraction, internal rotation and downward rotation of the scapula.
Nerve: Lateral and medial pectoral nerve, C5–T1.

Latissimus Dorsi

Origin: Spinous processes of T7–L5, iliac crest, thoracolumbar fascia, inferior angle of the scapula and lower 4 ribs.
Insertion: Bicipital groove.
Action: Depression, adducts, extends and internally rotates the humerus.
Nerve: Thoracodorsal nerve (C6–C8).

Deltoid

Origin: *Anterior Fibres* – Lateral third, anterior surface of the clavicle. *Middle Fibres* – Acromion process superior surface. *Posterior Fibres* – Spine of the scapula posterior border.
Insertion: Deltoid tuberosity of humerus.
Action: *Anterior Fibres* – flex and medially rotate shoulder. *Middle Fibres* – abduct shoulder. *Posterior Fibres* – extend and laterally rotate shoulder.
Nerve: Axillary nerve (C5–6).

Teres Major

Origin: Dorsal surface of the inferior angle of the scapula.
Insertion: Medial lip of intertubercular sulcus of humerus.
Action: Adducts, extends and medially rotates the shoulder.
Nerve: Lower subscapular nerve (C5–7).

Supraspinatus

> **Origin**: Supraspinatus fossa of the scapula.
> **Insertion**: Greater tuberosity of the humerus, superior facet.
> **Action**: Abducts shoulder 0–15 degrees, when the main agonist, then assists deltoid up to 90 degrees abduction.
> **Nerve**: Suprascapular nerve (C5–6).

Infraspinatus

> **Origin**: Infraspinatus fossa of scapula and infraspinatus fascia.
> **Insertion**: Posterior aspect of greater tuberosity of humerus and the shoulder joint capsule.
> **Action**: External rotation of the shoulder.
> **Nerve**: Suprascapular nerve (C5–C6).

Teres Minor

> **Origin**: Upper two-thirds of the lateral border of the scapula.
> **Insertion**: Inferior facet of the greater tubercle of the humerus. Lower fibres insert into the humerus directly below the inferior facet of the greater tubercle of the humerus.
> **Action**: External rotation of the shoulder.
> **Nerve**: Axillary nerve (C5–6).

Subscapularis

> **Origin**: Subscapular fossa on the costal surface of the scapula.
> **Insertion**: Lesser tuberosity of the humerus and the front of the shoulder joint capsule.
> **Action**: Internal rotation of the shoulder.
> **Nerve**: Suprascapular nerve (C5–6).

Coracobrachialis

> **Origin:** Apex of the coracoid process.
> **Insertion:** Medial border of the humerus.
> **Action:** Flexes and adducts the humerus. Assists internal rotation.
> **Nerve:** Musculocutaneous nerve (C5–7).

Elbow

Bicep Brachii

> **Origin:** *Short Head* – Apex of the coracoid process of the scapula. *Long Head* – Supraglenoid tubercle of the scapula.
> **Insertion:** Radial tuberosity and fascia of forearm via bicipital aponeurosis.
> **Action:** Elbow flexion of the elbow and forearm supination.
> **Nerve:** Musculocutaneous nerve (C5–7).

Brachialis

Origin: Distal anterior aspect of the humerus.
Insertion: Coronoid process and the ulnar tuberosity.
Action: Elbow flexion.
Nerve: Musculocutaneous nerve (C5–6).

Brachioradialis

Origin: Lateral supracondylar ridge and lateral intermuscular septum.
Insertion: Radius proximal to styloid process.
Action: Elbow flexion.
Nerve: Radial nerve (C5–6).

Pronator Teres

Origin: *Humeral Head* – medial epicondyle of the humerus via common flexor tendon, intermuscular septum and deep antebrachial fascia. *Ulnar Head* – Medial side of the coronoid process of the ulna.
Insertion: Middle of the lateral surface of the radius.
Action: Pronates the forearm and assists in elbow flexion.
Nerve: Median nerve (C6–7).

Triceps Brachii

Origin: *Long Head* – Infraglenoid tubercle of the scapula. *Lateral Head* – lateral and posterior surfaces of the humerus above the radial groove and lateral intermuscular septum. *Medial Head* – Posterior surfaces of the humerus below the radial groove and from and medial intermuscular septum.
Insertion: Posterior surface of the olecranon process of the ulna, capsule of the elbow joint and antebrachial fascia.
Action: Elbow and shoulder extension.
Nerve: Radial nerve (C6–8).

Anconeus

Origin: Dorsal side of the lateral epicondyle of the humerus.
Insertion: Olecranon of the ulna, along the proximal third of the posterior face of the ulna.
Action: Elbow extension.
Nerve: Radial nerve (C6–C8).

Pronator Quadratus

Origin: Lower quarter of anterior surface of ulna.
Insertion: Lower quarter of anterior surface of radius.
Action: Pronates forearm.
Nerve: Anterior osseous branch of median nerve (C7–8).

Supinator

> **Origin:** Lateral epicondyle of humerus, radial collateral ligament, annular ligament, supinator crest of ulna.
> **Insertion:** Lateral, posterior and anterior surfaces of proximal third of radius.
> **Action:** Forearm supination.
> **Nerve:** Posterior interosseous nerve (C7–8).

Wrist and Hand

Flexor Carpi Ulnaris

> **Origin:** *Humeral Head* – medial epicondyle of the humerus. Ulnar head – medial border of olecranon and upper two-thirds of border of ulna.
> **Insertion:** Pisiform bone, hook of hamate and base of 5th metacarpal.
> **Action:** Flexes and adducts the wrist.
> **Nerve:** Ulnar nerve (C7–T1).

Flexor Carpi Radialis

> **Origin:** Medial epicondyle of the humerus, lateral side of the forearm.
> **Insertion:** Bases of the second and third metacarpal bones.
> **Action:** Wrist flexion and abduction.
> **Nerve:** Median nerve (C6–7).

Palmaris Longus

> **Origin:** Medial epicondyle of the humerus via the common flexor tendon.
> **Insertion:** Palmar aponeurosis and flexor retinaculum at the wrist joint.
> **Action:** Wrist flexion.
> **Nerve:** Median nerve (C7–8).

Flexor Digitorum Superficialis

> **Origin:** *Humeroulnar head* – medial epicondyle via common flexor tendon, medial part or coronoid process of ulna, ulnar collateral ligament, intermuscular septa. Radial head – *upper two-thirds of anterior border of radius.*
> **Insertion:** Tendons divide and insert into sides of shaft of middle phalanx of 2nd–5th digits.
> **Action:** Wrist and finger flexion.
> **Nerve:** Median (C8–T1).

Flexor Digitorum Profundus

> **Origin:** Proximal half of anterior surface of ulna, interosseous membrane.
> **Insertion:** Palmar surfaces of distal phalanges of digits 2–5.
> **Action:** 2nd–5th metacarpophalangeal and interphalangeal joints flexion.
> **Nerve:** Digits 2–3 Median nerve. Digits 4–5 Ulnar nerve (C8, T1).

Flexor Pollicis Longus

> **Origin:** Anterior surface of radius and interosseous membrane.
> **Insertion:** Palmar surface of distal phalanx of thumb.
> **Action:** 1st metacarpophalangeal and interphalangeal joint (thumb) flexion.
> **Nerve:** Median nerve (anterior interosseous nerve C7–8).

Extensor Carpi Radialis Longus

> **Origin:** Lateral supracondylar ridge of humerus, lateral intermuscular septum of arm.
> **Insertion:** Posterior aspect of base of 2nd metacarpal.
> **Action:** Wrist extension and radial deviation.
> **Nerve:** Radial nerve (C5–C8).

Extensor Carpi Radialis Brevis

> **Origin:** Lateral epicondyle of humerus (common extensor tendon).
> **Insertion:** Posterior aspect of base of 3rd metacarpal.
> **Action:** Wrist joints: Wrist extension and radial deviation.
> **Nerve:** Radial nerve (C5– C6).

Extensor Carpi Ulnaris

> **Origin:** Lateral epicondyle of humerus, posterior border of ulna.
> **Insertion:** Base of 5th metacarpal.
> **Action:** Wrist joint: Wrist extension and radial deviation.
> **Nerve:** Posterior interosseous nerve (C7–8).

Extensor Digitorum

> **Origin:** Lateral epicondyle of humerus (common extensor tendon).
> **Insertion:** Extensor expansions of digits 2–5.
> **Action:** 2nd–5th metacarpophalangeal and interphalangeal joints extension.
> **Nerve:** Posterior interosseous nerve (C7–8).

Extensor Indicis

> **Origin:** Posterior surface of distal third of ulna and interosseus membrane.
> **Insertion:** Extensor expansion of index finger.
> **Action:** Extends all joints of index finger.
> **Nerve:** Posterior interosseous nerve (C7–8).

Extensor Digiti Minimi

> **Origin:** Lateral epicondyle of humerus (common extensor tendon).
> **Insertion:** Extensor expansion of little finger.
> **Action:** 5th metacarpophalangeal joint extension.
> **Nerve:** Posterior interosseous nerve (C7–8).

Extensor Pollicis Longus

> **Origin:** Posterior surface of middle third of ulna and interosseous membrane.
> **Insertion:** Posterior aspect of base of distal phalanx of thumb.
> **Action:** Extends interphalangeal and metacarpophalangeal joints of thumb.
> **Nerve:** Posterior interosseous nerve (C7–8).

Extensor Pollicis Brevis

> **Origin:** Posterior surface of distal third of radius and interosseous membrane.
> **Insertion:** Posterior aspect of base of proximal phalanx of thumb.
> **Action:** 1st Carpometacarpal and metacarpophalangeal joint extension.
> **Nerve:** Posterior interosseous nerve (C7–8).

Abductor Pollicis Longus

> **Origin:** Posterior surface of proximal half of radius, ulna and interosseous membrane.
> **Insertion:** Base of 1st metacarpal (trapezium).
> **Action:** Abducts and extends thumb at carpometacarpal joint.
> **Nerve:** Posterior interosseous nerve (C7–8).

Lumbricals

> **Origin:** Radial aspects of tendons of flexor digitorum profundus.
> **Insertion:** Dorsal aponeurosis of digits 2–5.
> **Action:** 2nd–5th Metacarpophalangeal joint flexion. 2nd–5th Interphalangeal joint extension.
> **Nerve:** Lumbricals 1–2 Median nerve (C8–T1). Lumbricals 3–4 Ulnar nerve (C8–T1).

Flexor Digiti Minimi Brevis

> **Origin:** Flexor retinaculum and hook of hamate.
> **Insertion:** Ulnar side of base of proximal phalanx of little finger.
> **Action:** Flexes 5th metacarpophalangeal joint.
> **Nerve:** Deep branch of ulnar nerve (C8–T1).

Interossei

> **Origin:** Ulnar side of 2nd metacarpal, Radial side of 4th–5th metacarpals.
> **Insertion:** Proximal phalanges and dorsal extensor expansion on ulnar side of index and radial side of ring and little fingers and to ulnar sesamoid of thumb.
> **Action:** Abduct from axis of 3rd phalanx. Flexes metacarpophalangeal joint while extending interphalangeal joints.
> **Nerve:** Deep branch of ulnar nerve (C8–T1).

Dorsal Interossei

> **Origin:** Bipennate from inner aspects of shafts of all metacarpals.
> **Insertion:** Proximal phalanges and dorsal extensor expansion on radial side of index and middle fingers and ulnar side of middle and ring fingers.

Action: Abducts from axis of middle finger. Flexes metacarpophalangeal joint while extending interphalangeal joints.

Nerve: Deep branch of ulnar nerve (T1).

Abductor Minimi Digiti

Origin: Pisiform bone, pisohamate ligament and flexor retinaculum.

Insertion: Ulnar side of base of proximal phalanx of little finger and extensor expansion.

Action: Abducts little finger at metacarpophalangeal joint.

Nerve: Deep branch of ulnar nerve (C8–T1).

Opponens Digiti Minimi

Origin: Flexor retinaculum and hook of hamate.

Insertion: Ulnar border of shaft of 5th metacarpal.

Action: Opposes carpometacarpal and metacarpophalangeal joints of the little finger.

Nerve: Deep branch of ulnar nerve (C8–T1).

Palmar Interossei

Origin: Anterior shafts of 2nd, 4th and 5th metacarpals.

Insertion: Proximal phalanges and dorsal extensor expansion on ulnar side of index and radial side of ring and little fingers and to ulnar sesamoid of thumb.

Action: Adduct to axis of middle finger. Flexes metacarpophalangeal joint while extending interphalangeal joints.

Nerve: Deep branch of ulnar nerve (T1).

Opponens Pollicis

Origin: Flexor retinaculum and tubercle of trapezium.

Insertion: Whole of radial border of 1st metacarpal.

Action: Opposes carpometacarpal and metacarpophalangeal joints of thumb.

Nerve: Median nerve (C8–T1).

Adductor Pollicis

Origin: *Oblique head* base of 2nd and 3rd metacarpals, trapezoid and capitate. *Transverse head* palmar border and shaft of 3rd metacarpal.

Insertion: Ulnar sesamoid then ulnar side of base of proximal phalanx and tendon of extensor pollicis longus.

Action: Adducts carpometacarpal joint of thumb.

Nerve: Deep branch of ulnar nerve (T1).

Abductor Pollicis Brevis

Origin: Tubercle of scaphoid and flexor retinaculum.

Insertion: Radial sesamoid of proximal phalanx of thumb and tendon of extensor pollicis longus.

Action: Abducts thumb at metacarpophalangeal and carpometacarpal joints.
Nerve: Median nerve (C8–T1).

Hip

Psoas Major

Origin: Transverse processes of L1–5, bodies of T12–L5 and intervertebral discs below bodies of T12–L4.
Insertion: Middle surface of lesser trochanter of femur.
Action: Flexes and laterally rotates femur.
Nerve: Anterior primary rami of L1–2.

Iliacus

Origin: Upper 2/3 of iliac fossa of ilium, internal lip of iliac crest, lateral aspect of sacrum.
Insertion: Lesser trochanter of femur.
Action: Flexes and externally rotates the femur.
Nerve: Femoral nerve (L2–3).

Rectus Femoris

Origin: Anterior inferior iliac spine (AIIS).
Insertion: Quadriceps tendon to insert at the patella and tibial tuberosity via patellar ligament.
Action: Hip flexion and knee extension.
Nerve: Femoral nerve (L2–4).

Sartorius

Origin: Anterior superior iliac spine (ASIS).
Insertion: Superomedial surface of the tibia.
Action: Hip flexion, abduction and lateral rotation.
Nerve: Femoral nerve.

Pectineus

Origin: Superior pubic ramus (pectineal line of pubis).
Insertion: Pectineal line of femur, linea aspera of femur.
Action: Hip flexion, adduction, external rotation and internal rotation.
Nerve: Femoral nerve (L2, L3) and obturator nerve (L2, L3).

Gluteus Maximus

Origin: Posterolateral surface of sacrum and coccyx. Gluteal surface of ilium. Thoracolumbar fascia and sacrotuberous ligament.
Insertion: Iliotibial tract. Gluteal tuberosity of femur.
Action: Hip extension, external rotation, abduction and adduction.
Nerve: Inferior gluteal nerve (L5–S2).

Semitendinosus

Origin: Ischial tuberosity.
Insertion: Proximal end of tibia below medial condyle (via pes anserinus).
Action: Hip extension and internal rotation. Knee flexion and internal rotation.
Nerve: Tibial portion of the sciatic nerve (L5–S2).

Semimembranosus

Origin: Ischial tuberosity.
Insertion: Medial condyle of tibia.
Action: Hip extension and internal rotation. Knee flexion and internal rotation.
Nerve: Sciatic nerve (L5–S2).

Biceps Femoris

Origin: *Long head* ischial tuberosity and sacrotuberous ligament. *Short head* linea aspera of femur and lateral supracondylar line of femur.
Insertion: Head of fibula.
Action: Hip extension and external rotation. Knee flexion and external rotation.
Nerve: *Long head* tibial division of sciatic nerve (L5–S2). *Short head* common fibular division of sciatic nerve (L5–S2).

Gluteus Medius

Origin: Gluteal surface of ilium between anterior and posterior gluteal lines.
Insertion: Lateral aspect of greater trochanter.
Action: Hip abduction and internal rotation.
Nerve: Superior gluteal nerve (L4–S1).

Gluteus Minimus

Origin: Outer surface of ilium between middle and inferior gluteal lines.
Insertion: Anterior surface of greater trochanter of femur.
Action: Abducts and medially rotates hip.
Nerve: Superior gluteal nerve (L4–S1).

Tensor Fascia Lata

Origin: Outer surface of anterior iliac crest between tubercle of the iliac crest and anterior superior iliac spine (ASIS).
Insertion: Iliotibial tract (anterior surface of lateral condyle of tibia).
Action: Hip internal rotation and abduction.
Nerve: Superior gluteal nerve (L4–S1).

Piriformis

> **Origin:** Anterior aspect of the sacrum at level S2–S4. Sacrotuberous ligament. Periphery of the greater sciatic notch.
> **Insertion:** Superiomedial aspect of the greater trochanter.
> **Action:** Lateral rotation of hip when extended. Abduction of hip when flexed.
> **Nerve:** Sacral plexus (L5–S2).

Adductor Magnus

> **Origin:** *Adductor portion* ischiopubic ramus. *Hamstring portion* lower outer quadrant of posterior surface of ischial tuberosity.
> **Insertion:** *Adductor portion* lower gluteal line and linea aspera. *Hamstring portion* adductor tubercle.
> **Action:** *Adductor portion* adducts and internally rotates hip. *Hamstring portion* extends hip.
> **Nerve:** *Adductor portion* posterior division of obturator nerve (L2–4). *Hamstring portion* tibial portion of sciatic (L4–S3).

Adductor Longus

> **Origin:** Body of pubis, inferior to pubic crest and lateral to the pubic symphysis.
> **Insertion:** Lower two-thirds of linea aspera (medial lip).
> **Action:** Hip adduction and internal rotation.
> **Nerve:** Obturator nerve (L2–L4).

Adductor Brevis

> **Origin:** Anterior body of pubis, inferior pubic ramus.
> **Insertion:** Linea aspera of femur (medial lip).
> **Action:** Hip flexion, adduction and external rotation.
> **Nerve:** Obturator nerve (L2–L3).

Gracilis

> **Origin:** Anterior body of pubis, inferior pubic ramus, ischial ramus.
> **Insertion:** Medial surface of proximal tibia (via pes anserinus).
> **Action:** Hip flexion and adduction. Knee joint flexion and medial rotation.
> **Nerve:** Obturator nerve (L2–L3).

Obturator Internus

> **Origin:** Anterior surface of the obturator membrane; bony boundaries of the obturator foramen.
> **Insertion:** Medial surface of greater trochanter of femur.
> **Action:** Hip external rotation.
> **Nerve:** Nerve to obturator internus (L5–S2).

Gemellus Superior

> **Origin:** Ischial spine.
> **Insertion:** Medial surface of greater trochanter of femur (via tendon of obturator internus).
> **Action:** Hip external rotation, abduction (from flexed hip); stabilises head of femur in acetabulum.
> **Nerve:** Nerve to obturator internus (L5–S1).

Gemellus Inferior

> **Origin:** Ischial tuberosity.
> **Insertion:** Medial surface of greater trochanter via tendon of obturator internus.
> **Action:** Hip external rotation and abduction (from flexed hip), stabilises head of femur in acetabulum.
> **Nerve:** Nerve to quadratus femoris (L4–S1).

Quadratus Femoris

> **Origin:** Ischial tuberosity.
> **Insertion:** Intertrochanteric crest of femur.
> **Action:** Hip external rotation and stabilises head of femur in acetabulum.
> **Nerve:** Nerve to quadratus femoris (L4–S1).

Obturator Externus

> **Origin:** Anterior surface of obturator membrane, bony boundaries of obturator foramen.
> **Insertion:** Trochanteric fossa of femur.
> **Action:** Hip external rotation and abduction (from flexed hip); Stabilises head of femur in acetabulum.
> **Nerve:** Obturator nerve (L3–4).

Knee

Semitendinosus – See Hip.
Semimembranosus – See Hip.
Biceps Femoris – See Hip.
Gastrocnemius

> **Origin:** *Lateral head* – posterolateral aspect of lateral condyle of the femur. *Medial head* – posterior surface of medial femoral condyle, popliteal surface of femoral shaft.
> **Insertion:** Posterior surface of the calcaneus via the Achilles tendon.
> **Action:** Plantar flexion and knee flexion.
> **Nerve:** Tibial nerve (S1–2).

Gracilis

> **Origin:** Anterior body of pubis, inferior pubic ramus, ischial ramus.
> **Insertion:** Medial surface of proximal tibia (via pes anserinus).
> **Action:** Hip flexion and adduction. Knee flexion and medial rotation.
> **Nerve:** Obturator nerve (L2–3).

Sartorius – See Hip.
Plantaris

> **Origin:** Lateral supracondylar line of femur, oblique popliteal ligament of knee.
> **Insertion:** Posterior surface of calcaneus via Achilles tendon.
> **Action:** Plantar flexion and knee flexion.
> **Nerve:** Tibial nerve (S1–2).

Popliteus

> **Origin:** Lateral femoral condyle, Posterior horn of lateral meniscus of knee joint.
> **Insertion:** Posterior surface of proximal tibia.
> **Action:** Unlocks extended knee by lateral rotation of femur on tibia.
> **Nerve:** Tibial nerve (L5–S2).

Rectus Femoris – See Hip.
Vastus Lateralis

> **Origin:** Upper inter-trochanteric line, base of greater trochanter, lateral linea aspera, lateral supracondylar ridge and lateral intermuscular septum.
> **Insertion:** Lateral quadriceps tendon to patella, via ligamentum patellae into tibia tubercle.
> **Action:** Extends knee.
> **Nerve:** Posterior division of femoral nerve (L3–4).

Vastus Intermedius

> **Origin:** Upper two-thirds of anterior and lateral surfaces of the femur and the intermuscular septum.
> **Insertion:** Quadriceps tendon to patella via ligamentum patellae into tibia tubercle.
> **Action:** Extends knee.
> **Nerve:** Posterior division of femoral nerve (L3–4).

Vastus Medialis

> **Origin:** Lower intertrochanteric line, spiral line, medial linea aspera and medial intermuscular septum.
> **Insertion:** Medial quadriceps tendon to patella and directly into medial patella, via ligamentum patellae into tubercle of tibia.
> **Action:** Extends knee. Stabilises patella.
> **Nerve:** Posterior division of femoral nerve (L3–4).

Tensor Fascia Lata – See Hip.

Ankle

Gastrocnemius – See Knee.
Soleus

> **Origin:** Soleal line, medial border of tibia, head of fibula, posterior border of fibula.
> **Insertion:** Posterior surface of calcaneus via Achilles tendon.
> **Action:** Plantar flexion.
> **Nerve:** Tibial nerve (S1–2).

Plantaris – See Knee.
Peroneus Longus

> **Origin:** Upper two-thirds of lateral shaft of fibula, head of fibula and superior tibiofibular joint.
> **Insertion:** Plantar aspect of base of 1st metatarsal and medial cuneiform, passing deep to long plantar ligament.
> **Action:** Plantarflexion and eversion. Supports lateral longitudinal and transverse arches.
> **Nerve:** Superficial peroneal nerve (L5–S1).

Tibialis Posterior

> **Origin:** Upper half of posterior shaft of tibia and upper half of fibula between medial nerve crest and interosseous border and interosseous membrane.
> **Insertion:** Tuberosity of navicular bone and all tarsal bones (except talus) and spring ligament.
> **Action:** Plantarflexion and inversion. Supports medial longitudinal arch of foot.
> **Nerve:** Tibial nerve (L4–5).

Flexor Digitorum Longus

> **Origin:** Posterior shaft of tibia below soleal line and by broad aponeurosis from fibula.
> **Insertion:** Base of distal phalanges of lateral four toes.
> **Action:** Flexes distal phalanges of lateral four toes and foot at ankle. Supports lateral longitudinal arch.
> **Nerve:** Tibial nerve (S1–2).

Flexor Hallucis Longus

> **Origin:** Lower two-thirds of posterior fibula between median crest and posterior border, lower intermuscular septum and aponeurosis of flexor digitorum longus.
> **Insertion:** Base of distal phalanx of big toe and slips to medial of flexor digitorum longus.
> **Action:** Flexes distal phalanx of hallux, Plantarflexion, Inversion supports medial longitudinal arch.
> **Nerve:** Tibial nerve (S2–3).

Peroneus Brevis

> **Origin:** Lower two-thirds lateral shaft of fibula.
> **Insertion:** Tuberosity of base of 5th metatarsal.
> **Action:** Plantarflexion and eversion. Supports lateral longitudinal arch.
> **Nerve:** Superficial peroneal nerve (L5–S1).

Tibialis Anterior

> **Origin:** Lateral surface of tibia, interosseous membrane.
> **Insertion:** Medial cuneiform bone, base of metatarsal bone 1.
> **Action:** Dorsiflexion and inversion.
> **Nerve:** Deep fibular nerve (L4–5).

Extensor Digitorum Longus

> **Origin:** Upper two-thirds of anterior shaft of fibula, interosseous membrane and superior tibiofibular joint.
> **Insertion:** Extensor expansion of lateral four toes.
> **Action:** Extends toes and dorsiflexion.
> **Nerve:** Deep peroneal nerve (L5–S1).

Extensor Hallucis Longus

> **Origin:** Middle third of medial surface of fibula, interosseous membrane.
> **Insertion:** Base of distal phalanx of hallux.
> **Action:** Extends hallux and dorsiflexion. Inverts foot and tightens subtalar joints
> **Nerve:** Deep fibular nerve (L5–S1).

Peroneus Tertius

> **Origin:** Third quarter of anterior shaft of fibula.
> **Insertion:** Shaft and base of 5th metatarsal.
> **Action:** Dorsiflexion and eversion.
> **Nerve:** Deep peroneal nerve (L5–S1).

Toes

Flexor Digitorum Longus – See Ankle.
Flexor Digitorum Accessorius

> **Origin:** Medial surface of calcaneus bone, lateral process of calcaneal tuberosity.
> **Insertion:** Tendon of flexor digitorum longus.
> **Action:** Flexion of the 2nd–5th metatarsophalangeal joints.
> **Nerve:** Lateral plantar nerve (S1–S3).

Flexor Digitorum Brevis

> **Origin:** Medial process of posterior calcaneal tuberosity.
> **Insertion:** Middle phalanges of digits 2–5.
> **Action:** Flexes lateral four toes. Supports medial and lateral longitudinal arches.
> **Nerve:** Medial plantar nerve (S1–2).

Flexor Hallucis Longus – See Ankle.
Flexor Hallucis Brevis

> **Origin:** Tibialis posterior tendon, medial and lateral cuneiform and cuboid.
> **Insertion:** Lateral and medial aspects of base of proximal phalanx of hallux.

Action: Flexes metatarsophalangeal joint of hallux. Supports medial longitudinal arch.
Nerve: Medial plantar nerve (S1–2).

Flexor Digiti Minimi Brevis

Origin: Base of 5th metatarsal, long plantar ligament.
Insertion: Base of proximal phalanx of 5th digit.
Action: 5th metatarsophalangeal joint flexion.
Nerve: Lateral plantar nerve (S2–3).

Interossei

Origin: Bipennate from inner aspects of shafts of all metatarsals.
Insertion: Bases of proximal phalanges and dorsal extensor expansions of medial side of 2nd toe and lateral sides of 2nd, 3rd and 4th toes.
Action: Abduct 2nd, 3rd and 4th toes from axis of 2nd toe. Assist lumbricals in extending interphalangeal joints while flexing metatarsal phalangeal joints.
Nerve: Lateral plantar nerve (S2–3).

Lumbricals

Origin: Tendons of flexor digitorum longus.
Insertion: Medial bases of proximal phalanges and extensor expansion of digits 2–5.
Action: Flexion and adduction 2nd–5th metatarsophalangeal joints. Extension 2nd–5th Interphalangeal joints.
Nerve: *Lumbrical 1* – Medial plantar nerve (S2–3). *Lumbricals 2–4* – Lateral plantar nerve (S2–3).

Abductor Hallucis

Origin: Medial process of calcaneal tuberosity, flexor retinaculum, plantar aponeurosis.
Insertion: Base of proximal phalanx of hallux.
Action: Abduction and flexion 1st metatarsophalangeal joint. Support of longitudinal arch of foot.
Nerve: Medial plantar nerve (S1–S3).

Extensor Hallucis Longus – See Ankle.
Extensor Digitorum Longus – See Ankle.
Extensor Digitorum Brevis

Origin: Superolateral surface of calcaneus, interosseous talocalcaneal ligament; stem of inferior extensor retinaculum.
Insertion: 2nd–4th Extensor digitorum longus tendons.
Action: Extension of 2nd–4th distal interphalangeal joints.
Nerve: Deep peroneal nerve (L5–S1).

Abductor Digiti Minimi

Origin: Calcaneal tuberosity, plantar aponeurosis.
Insertion: Base of 5th proximal phalanx, 5th metatarsal.

Action: Flexion and abduction 5th metatarsophalangeal joint. Supports longitudinal arch of foot.

Nerve: Lateral plantar nerve (S1–3).

Dorsal Interossei

Origin: Opposing sides of 1st–5th metatarsal bones.

Insertion: 1st medial base of proximal phalanx of digit. 2nd– th – lateral bases of proximal phalanges and extensor expansion of 2nd–4th digits.

Action: Flexion and abduction 2nd–4th metatarsophalangeal joints. Extension 2nd–4th Interphalangeal joints.

Nerve: Lateral plantar nerve (S2–3).

Adductor Hallucis

Origin: *Oblique head* – bases of 2nd–4th metatarsal, cuboid, lateral cuneiform, fibularis longus tendon. *Transverse head* – plantar metatarsophalangeal ligaments of toes 3–5, deep transverse metatarsal ligaments of toes 3–5.

Insertion: Lateral aspect of base of proximal phalanx of hallux.

Action: Adduction and flexion 1st metatarsophalangeal joint. Support of longitudinal and transverse arches of foot.

Nerve: Lateral plantar nerve (S2–3).

Plantar Interossei

Origin: Medial aspects of 3rd–5th metatarsals.

Insertion: Medial bases of proximal phalanges and extensor expansion of digits 3–5.

Action: Flexion and adduction 3rd–5th metatarsophalangeal joints. Extension 3rd– th Interphalangeal joints.

Nerve: Lateral plantar nerve (S2–3) (Adapted from [1–2, 4–5]).

Joints

A joint is the articulation between bones in the body which connect the skeletal system. They are constructed to allow for different degrees and types of movement (Figure 1.5, Table 1.1) [1, 3].

Ligaments

Ligaments can be defined as short bands of tough, flexible fibrous connective tissue which connect bone to bone to form joints (Table 1.2).

Frontalis

Temporalis

Sternocleidomastoid
Platysma
Sternohyoid
Trapezius

Deltoid

Pectoralis major

Serratus anterior
Biceps
External abdominal oblique
Rectus abdominus

Linea alba
Tendinous inscription

Brachioradialis

Inguinal ligament

Tensor fasciae latae
Adductor longus

Sartorius

Rectus femoris
Vastus lateralis

Vastus medialis

Patellar ligament

Tibialis anterior

Gastrocnemius

Muscles of the Body, Anterior View

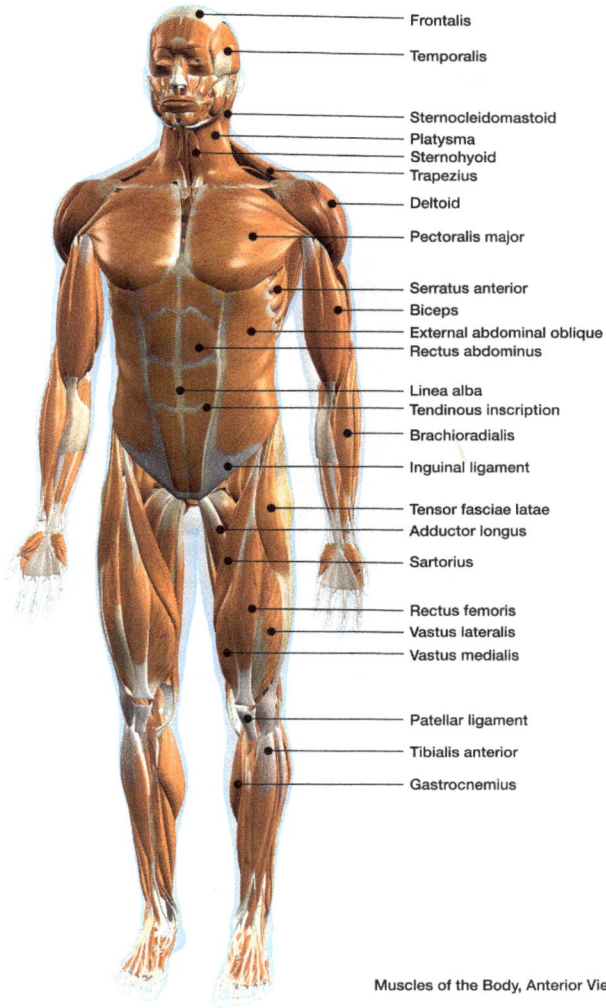

FIGURE 1.3   Muscles of the body. Anterior view.

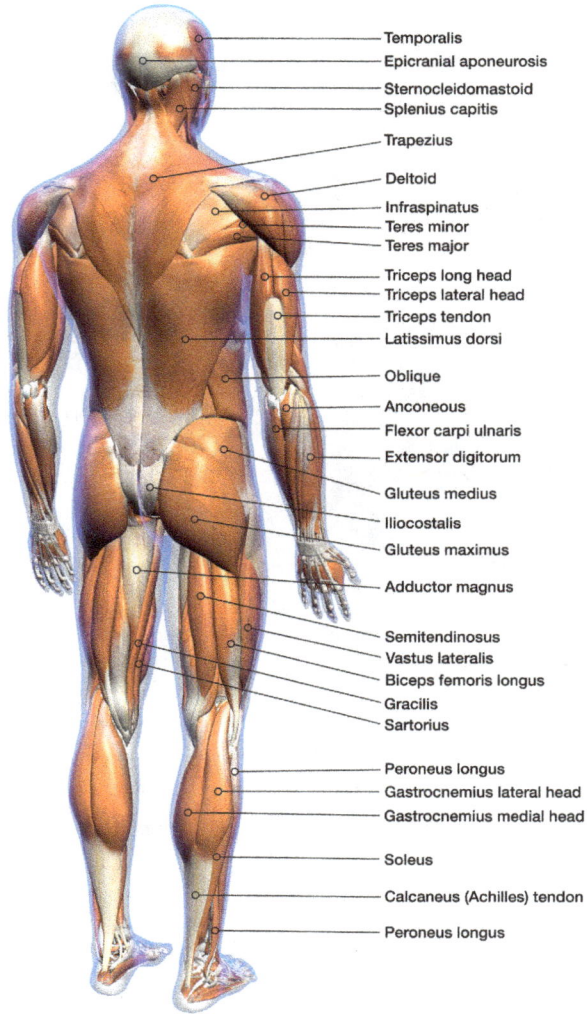

Temporalis
Epicranial aponeurosis
Sternocleidomastoid
Splenius capitis
Trapezius
Deltoid
Infraspinatus
Teres minor
Teres major
Triceps long head
Triceps lateral head
Triceps tendon
Latissimus dorsi
Oblique
Anconeous
Flexor carpi ulnaris
Extensor digitorum
Gluteus medius
Iliocostalis
Gluteus maximus
Adductor magnus
Semitendinosus
Vastus lateralis
Biceps femoris longus
Gracilis
Sartorius
Peroneus longus
Gastrocnemius lateral head
Gastrocnemius medial head
Soleus
Calcaneus (Achilles) tendon
Peroneus longus

FIGURE 1.4   Muscles of the body. Posterior view.

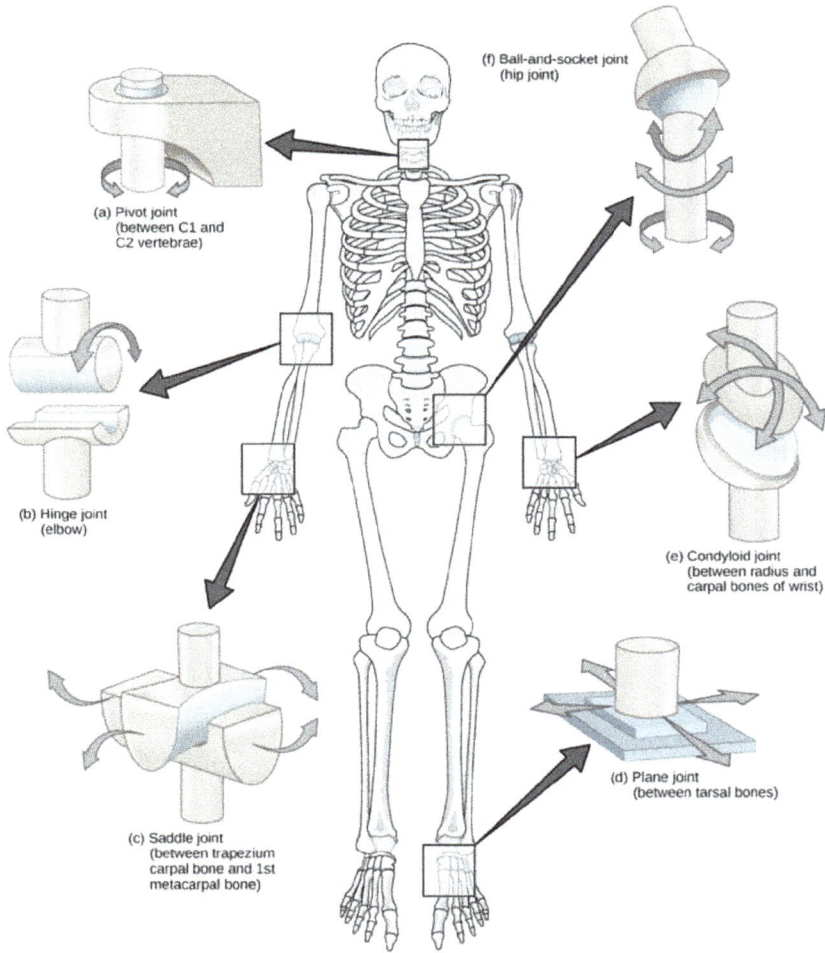

FIGURE 1.5 Types of joints.

TABLE 1.1 Joints within the body and normal range of movement values

Joint	Anatomical joint name	Anatomical joint	Normal ROM values
Facet Joints	Zygapophyseal or Apophyseal joints	Plane joint	N/A
Spine	Vertebral bodies	Secondary cartilaginous joints	*Cervical Spine* Flexion = 80–90° Extension = 70° Lateral flexion = 20–46° Rotation = 80–90°
			Lumbar Spine Flexion = 50–60° Extension = 20–25° Lateral flexion = 20–25°

(*continued*)

TABLE 1.1 Cont.

Joint	Anatomical joint name	Anatomical joint	Normal ROM values
Shoulder	Glenohumeral joint	Ball & socket joint	Flexion = 180° Extension = 45/60° Abduction = 150/160° Adduction = 30–50° Horizontal abduction = 90° Horizontal adduction = 50° External rot = 90° Internal rot = 70/90°
Elbow	Proximal radioulnar joint	Pivot joint	Supination = 85° Pronation = 70°
Elbow	Humeroradial joint	Pivot joint	Flexion = 150° Extension = 0–5°
Elbow	Humeroulnar joint	Hinge joint	Flexion = 150° Extension = 0–5°
Wrist	Radiocarpal joint	Condyloid joint	Flexion = 50° Extension = 30–40° Radial deviation = 30° Ulna deviation = 30°
Wrist	Metacarpophalangeal joint	Condyloid joint	Flexion = 50–60° Extension = 0–10° Abduction = 15° Adduction = 15°
Fingers	Interphalangeal joints	Uniaxial hinge joints	Flexion = 90° Extension = 5°
Hip	Acetabulofemoral joint	Ball & socket joint	Flexion = 110–130° Extension = 30–40° Abduction = 45–50° Adduction = 20–30° External rotation = 45° Internal rotation = 40°
Knee	Patellofemoral joint	Plane joint	
Knee	Tibiofemoral joint	Biaxial hinge joint	Flexion = 140–150° Extension = 0–5°
Ankle	Talocrural joint	Uniaxial hinge joint	Plantarflexion = 45–50° Dorsiflexion = 20°
Ankle	Subtalar joint	Plane joint	Inversion = 20–30° Eversion = 15–20° Pronation = 5° Supination = 20°
Foot	Metatarsophalangeal	Condyloid joint	Flexion = 45° Extension = 70°
Foot	Interphalangeal joints	Uniaxial hinge joint	Flexion = 90° Extension = 0°

TABLE 1.2 Ligaments within the body and their role

Joint	Ligament	Origin	Insertion	Role
Spine	Supraspinous	C7	Sacrum	Limits flexion
	Ligamentum Flavum	Runs between the lamina from the axis to sacrum		Limits flexion
	Anterior Longitudinal	Front of the vertebral body to the front of the annulus fibrosis	Upper & lower edges of each vertebral body	Limits extension & reinforces front of annulus fibrosis
	Posterior Longitudinal	Runs in the spinal canal attaching to the vertebral bodies & vertebral discs		Limits flexion & reinforces back of annulus fibrosis
	Alar	Odontoid process	Medial aspect of the occipital condyles	Limits head rotation & lateral flexion
	Anterior Atlantoaxial	Strong membrane, fixed, above to the lower border of the anterior arch of the atlas; below, to the front of the body of the axis		Limits extension
	Posterior Atlantoaxial	Broad thin membrane attached, above, to the lower border of the posterior arch of the atlas; below, to the upper edges of the lamina of the axis		Limits flexion
	Ligamentum Nuchae	External occipital protuberance on the skull & median nuchal line	Spinous process of C7	Limits flexion
	Interspinous	Root of each spinous process	Apex of each spinous process	Limits flexion
	Intertransverse	Interposed between the transverse processes		Limits lateral flexion
	Iliolumbar	Tip of the transverse process of the fifth lumbar vertebra	Posterior part of the inner lip of the iliac crest	Stability
	Anterior Sacroiliac	Anterior surface of the lateral part of the sacrum	Margin of the auricular surface of the ilium & to the preauricular sulcus	Stability
	Posterior Sacroiliac	*Upper Part*: 1st & 2nd transverse tubercles on the back of the sacrum. *Lower Part*: 3rd transverse tubercle of the back of the sacrum	*Upper Part*: tuberosity of the ilium. *Lower Part*: posterior superior spine of the ilium	Stability
	Sacrospinous	Lateral margin of the inferior sacrum	Ischial spine	Stability & resisting external rotation forces of the pelvis
	Sacrotuberous	Sacrum, coccyx, ilium & sacroiliac joint capsule	Medial ischial tuberosity & additional fibres extend to the ischial ramus	Stability

(continued)

TABLE 1.2 Cont.

Joint	Ligament	Origin	Insertion	Role
Shoulder	Coracoacromial	*Conoid ligament:* knuckle of the coracoid process of the scapula. *Trapezoid ligament:* Trapezoid ridge on the coracoid process of the scapula	Undersurface of the clavicle (around the conoid tubercle). Underside of the clavicle (to the trapezoid ridge)	Limits superior displacement of the HH from the glenoid
	Coracohumeral	Lateral border of the coracoid process	Greater tubercle of the humerus, blending with the supraspinatus tendon	Limits flexion, extension, inferior & posterior translation of HH
	Transverse Humeral	Bridging the lesser and greater tubercle of the humerus	Superior to the epiphysial line	Limits subluxation of LHB
	Superior Glenohumeral	Glenoid rim	Anatomical neck of humerus	Limits external rotation & inferior translation of the HH
	Middle Glenohumeral	Glenoid rim	Anatomical neck of humerus	Limits external rotation & anterior translation of the HH
	Inferior Glenohumeral	Glenoid rim	Lesser tuberosity of the humerus	*Anterior portion:* Limits external rotation, superior & anterior translation of the HH. *Posterior portion:* Limits internal rotation & anterior translation of HH
Elbow	Radial Collateral	Lateral epicondyle of the humerus	Lateral part of the annular ligament, the radius and also the ulnar	Lateral stabiliser & resists varus stress
	Ulnar Collateral	Anterior inferior surface of the medial epicondyle	Proximal ulnar cartilage	Medial stabiliser & resists valgus stress
	Annular	Runs around the radial head form the anterior & the posterior margin of the radial notch		Stabilises radial head during supinationm& pronation
Wrist	Ulnar Collateral	Styloid process of the ulna	Medial side of the triquetral bone, pisiform & flexor retinaculum	Limits Radial deviation
	Radial Collateral	Styloid process of the radius	Scaphoid bone	Limits ulnar deviation
	Dorsal Radiocollateral	Radius	Both rows of carpal bones	Stability. Ensure hand follows the forearm during pronation
	Palmar Radiocollateral	Radius	Both rows of carpal bones	Stability. Ensure hand follows the forearm during supination

Hip	Iliofemoral	Anterior Inferior Iliac Spine (AIIS)	Intertrochanteric line of the femur	Limits hyperextension
	Pubofemoral	Iliopubic ramus, superior pubic ramus & obturator crest of the pubic bone	Intertrochanteric line, blending with the fibrous layer of the joint capsule & the medial band of the iliofemoral ligament	Limits excess abduction & extension
	Ischiofemoral	Anterior inferior iliac spine (AIIS) & the rim of the acetabulum	Intertrochanteric line on the anterior side of the femoral head	Limits excess extension
Knee	Anterior Cruciate	Medial wall of the lateral femoral condyle	Middle of the intercondylar area	Stability & Limits anterior translation of tibia
	Posterior Cruciate	Anterolateral aspect of the medial femoral condyle within the notch	Posterior aspect of the tibial plateau	Stability & limits posterior translation of tibia
	Medial Collateral	Medial femoral condyle	Medial aspect of the shaft of the tibia	Stability & limits valgus stress
	Lateral Collateral	Lateral femoral epicondyle	Joins the bicep femoris tendon before attaching to head of fibula	Stability & limits varus stress
Ankle	Anterior Talofibular	Anterior margin of lateral malleolus	Neck of talus	Limits anterior displacement of the talus. Inversion in plantarflexion
	Calcaneofibular	Lateral malleolus	Lateral surface of calcaneus	Stability during dorsiflexion. Limits Inversion of the calcaneus. Limits Talar tilt into inversion
	Posterior Talofibular	Malleolar fossa of fibula	Lateral tubercle of talus	Limits posterior displacement of the talus
	Bifurcate	*Calcaneocuboid ligament*: anterior aspect of the superior surface of the calcaneus. *Calcaneocuboid ligament*: anterior aspect of the superior surface of the calcaneus	Dorsomedial surface of the cuboid bone / Dorsolateral surface of the navicular bone.	Stabilises the calcaneocuboid joint
	Anterior Tibiotalar	Medial malleolus	Head of talus	Stability. Control plantarflexion & Eversion
	Posterior Tibiotalar	Medial malleolus	Talus posteriorly	Control dorsiflexion
	Tibionavicular	Medial malleolus	Dorsomedial aspect of navicular	Stability
	Tibiocalcaneal	Medial malleolus	Sustentaculum tali	Stability

*HH = Humeral Head. *LHB = Long Head of Bicep.

Nervous System

The nervous system is a complex collection of nerves and specialised cells known as neurons that transmit signals between different parts of the body. It is essentially the body's electrical wiring. Structurally, the nervous system has two components: the central nervous system and the peripheral nervous system.

The **central nervous system** (CNS) controls most functions of the body and mind. It consists of two parts, the brain and the spinal cord.

The **peripheral nervous system** refers to the parts of the nervous system that are outside the CNS. Its function is to relay information to and from your CNS. The peripheral nerves transmit voluntary and involuntary actions, such as: sympathetic nervous system (fight or flight) and the parasympathetic nervous system (rest and digest) (Figure 1.6).

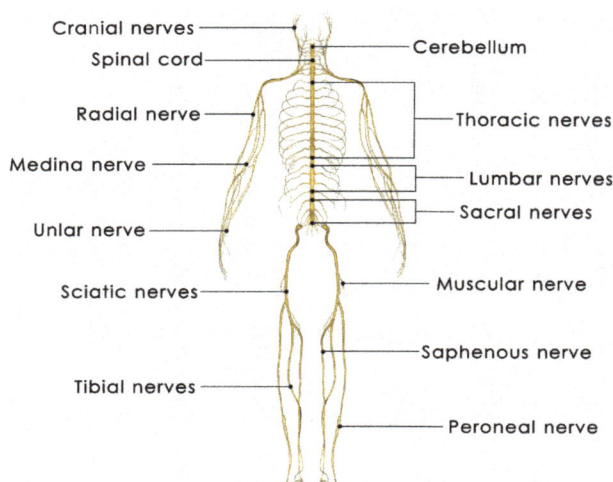

FIGURE 1.6 The peripheral nervous system.

Vascular and Lymphatic System

The vascular system, also known as the circulatory system, consists of the vessels that transport blood and lymph through the body. The arteries and veins transport blood throughout the body, delivering oxygen and nutrients to the body's tissues and removing tissue waste matter.

The lymphatic system helps protect and maintain the fluid environment of the body by filtering and draining lymph away from each body region.

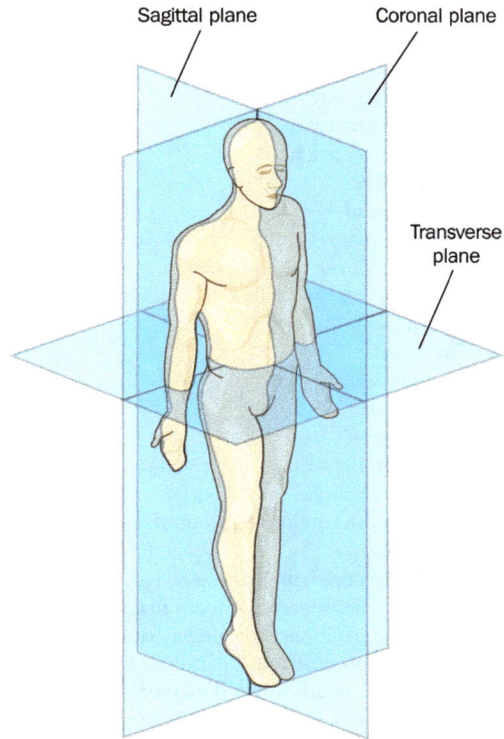

FIGURE 1.7 The three planes of movement.

Planes of Movement

Movements of the human body are often described in terms of the 'plane' in which they pass through. There are three planes of the human body, coronal, sagittal and transverse (Figure 1.7).

Anatomical Terms of Movement

Anatomical terms of movement are used to describe the actions of muscles upon the skeleton. Muscles contract to produce movement at joints, and the subsequent movements can be precisely described using this terminology. The terms (Table 1.3) used assume that the body begins in the anatomical position.

TABLE 1.3 Clinical terminology and their meanings

Anterior	Front of the body
Posterior	Back of the body
Inferior	Below or towards feet
Superior	Above or towards head
Caudad	Towards feet
Cephalad	Towards head
Midline	An imaginary vertical line that divides the body equally down the middle
Lateral	Being away from the midline
Medial	Being towards the midline
Palmar surface of hand	The palm
Ventral	The palm
Dorsum of hand	Back of hand
Plantar surface of foot	Sole of foot
Dorsum of foot	Top of foot
Deep	Away from the surface of the body
Superficial	Close to the surface of the body
Flexion	Flexion is the bending of a joint so as to bring together the parts it connects
Extension	Extension is the straightening of a joint
Abduction	Abduction describes movement that is away from the midline of the body
Adduction	Adduction describes movement that is towards the midline of the body
Circumduction	A circular movement of a part. This is a combination of flexion, abduction, extension, adduction and rotation
Rotation	Movement of a bone around a longitudinal axis. Medial rotation is movement in which the anterior aspect of a limb turns towards the midline. Lateral rotation is movement in which the anterior aspect of a limb turns away from the mid line
Pronation	When in the anatomical position the forearm is rotated so that the palm of the hand faces backwards. If the elbow is flexed so that the forearm is horizontal the palm of the hand is turned to face downwards
Supination	The opposite of pronation. The palm of the hand is turned to face forwards of upwards if the forearm is horizontal
Inversion	Turning inwards of the plantar aspect of the foot
Eversion	Turning outwards of the plantar aspect of the foot
Dorsiflexion	A movement of the ankle which pulls the toes and foot up towards the body
Plantarflexion	Pointing of the toes and foot away from the body
Protraction	To move forwards (this term is used only in relationship to the shoulder and the jaw)
Retraction	To move backwards (this term is used only in relationship to the shoulder and the jaw)
Prone	Lying or positioned on the tummy
Supine	Lying or positioned on the back

References

1. Palastanga, N., & Soames, R. (2019). *Anatomy and human movement: Structure and function* (7th ed.). London: Elsevier.
2. Adds, P. J., & Sharsavari, S. (2012). *The musculoskeletal system.* London: Informa Healthcare.
3. Magee, D. J. (2013). *Orthopaedic physical assessment* (6th ed.). London: Elsevier.
4. Muscolino, J. E. (2012). *Know the body: Muscle, bone and palpation essentials.* Maryland Heights, MO: Elsevier.
5. Hansen, J. T. (2014). *Netter's clinical anatomy* (3rd ed.). Philadelphia, PA: Elsevier.

2

MUSCULOSKELETAL ASSESSMENT

Mark Richardson

Muscle Innervation

Each skeletal muscle within the body is innervated by a motor neuron but may also innervate other muscle fibres (Table 2.1, 2.2). A motor unit consists of all the fibres innervated by the same motor neuron. Groups of motor units often work together to coordinate a muscle contraction for both the upper limb and lower limb [1].

TABLE 2.1 Musculoskeletal muscle innervation chart of the upper limb

Innervation of the muscles of the upper limb				
T1	C8	C7	C6	C5

- Supraspinatus
- Infraspinatus
- Pectoralis major (upper)
- Deltoid
- Serratus anterior
- Rhomboid major & minor
- Supinator
- Biceps
- Brachioradialis
- Pronator teres
- Pectoralis minor
- Pectoralis major (lower)
- Triceps
- Extensor carpi radialis, longus & brevis
- Flexor carpi radialis
- Extensor digitorum
- Flexor carpi ulnaris
- Extensor digiti minimi
- Extensor carpi ulnaris
- Extensor pollicis longus
- Abductor pollicis longus
- Extensor pollicis brevis
- Extensor indicis
- Flexor digitorum superficialis
- Flexor digitorum profundus
- Adductor pollicis
- Flexor pollicis brevis
- Opponens pollicis
- Interossei
- Abductor pollicis brevis
- Lumbricals

Legend:
- Shoulder muscles
- Upper arm muscles
- Lower arm muscles
- Intrinsic hand muscles

TABLE 2.2 Musculoskeletal muscle innervation chart of the lower limb

Innervation of the muscles of the lower limb

Muscle	L4	L5	S1	S2
Gluteus maximus		X	X	X
Gluteus medius	X	X	X	
Gluteus minimus	X	X	X	
Tensor fascia latae	X	X	X	
Piriformis			X	X
Obturator internus		X	X	X
Superior gemellus		X	X	X
Inferior gemellus	X	X	X	
Quadratus femoris	X	X	X	
Adductor magnus	X	X		
Semitendinosus		X	X	
Semimembranosus		X	X	
Bicep femoris (long head)		X	X	X
Bicep Femoris (short head)		X	X	
Tibialis anterior	X	X	X	
Extensor digitorum longus	X	X	X	
Peroneus tertius	X	X	X	
Extensor halluces longus	X	X	X	
Peroneus longus	X	X	X	
Peroneus brevis	X	X	X	
Gastrocnemius			X	X
Soleus			X	X
Plantaris	X	X	X	
Popliteus		X	X	
Tibialis posterior		X	X	
Flexor digitorum longus		X	X	
Flexor halluces longus		X	X	X
Extensor hallucis brevis		X	X	
Extensor digitorum brevis		X	X	
Abductor hallucis		X	X	
Flexor halluces brevis		X	X	
Adductor hallucis			X	X
Flexor digitorum brevis		X	X	
Quadratus plantae			X	X
Flexor digiti minimi			X	X
Abductor digiti minimi			X	X
First lumbrical		X	X	
Lateral three lumbricals			X	X
Interossei			X	X

Legend:
- Buttock & hip muscles
- Thigh muscles
- Lower leg muscles
- Intrinsic foot muscles

Strength Testing

Manual Muscle Test (MMT)

An assessment of muscle strength is typically performed as part of a patient's objective assessment and is an important component of the physical exam that can reveal information about neurologic deficits. It is used to evaluate weakness and can be effective in differentiating true weakness from imbalance or poor endurance. It may be referred to as motor testing, muscle strength grading, manual muscle testing or any other synonym.

The most common way to assess muscle strength is by using the Medical Research Council strength scale (also known as the Oxford Scale, Table 2.3)

TABLE 2.3 Manual muscle test grading criteria

Manual Muscle Testing (MMT) Scores

Score	Description
0	No palpable or visible muscle contraction
1	Palpable or visible contraction but no motion
2–	Partial ROM, gravity eliminated
2	Full ROM, gravity eliminated
2+	Gravity eliminated/slight resistance
3–	> 1/2 but < Full ROM, against gravity
3	Full ROM against gravity
3+	Full ROM against gravity, slight resistance
4–	Full ROM against gravity, mild resistance
4	Full ROM against gravity, moderate resistance
4+	Full ROM against gravity, almost full resistance
5	Normal, maximal resistance

Brake Test

Isometric test, testing the muscle at mid-range, then slowly increase the pressure. The test is quicker to perform but less informative (Table 2.4).

TABLE 2.4 Brake test grading criteria

Brake Test

Strong & painless	Normal response suggesting injury is not neuromuscular
Strong & painful	Indicating a lesion in a muscle or tendon
Weak & painless	Indicating a nerve or musculotendinous rupture
Weak & painful	Indicating serious injury that could range from fracture to unstable joint

Hypermobility

Hypermobility is the term used to describe the ability to move joints beyond the normal range of movement. The Beighton hypermobility score (Figure 2.1) and Brighton criteria (Table 2.5) are both diagnostic criteria for benign joint hypermobility syndrome.

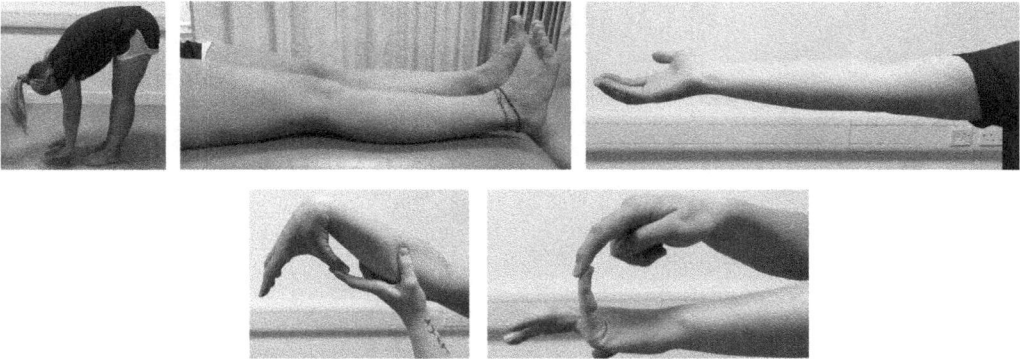

FIGURE 2.1   The five tests needed to be completed for the Beighton hypermobility score.

Beighton Hypermobility Score

A positive Beighton score for adults is 5 out of 9 possible points. For children a positive score is at least 6 out of 9 points (Figure 2.1).

TABLE 2.5 Brighton criteria

Major Criteria
>Beighton score of >4
>Arthralgia for longer than 3 months in 4 or more joints

Minor Criteria
>Beighton score of 1, 2 or 3
>Arthralgia (>3-month duration) or spondylosis, spondylolysis, spondylolisthesis
>Dislocation or subluxation in more than on joint or in 1 joint or on more than 1 occasion
>3 or more soft tissue lesions (e.g. epicondylitis, tenosynovitis, bursitis)
>Marfanoid habitus (tall, slim, span greater than height (>1.03 ratio), upper segment less than lower
>>segment (<0.89 ratio), arachnodactyly
>Skin striae, hyperextensibility, thin skin or abnormal scarring
>Ocular signs: drooping eyelids, myopia, antimongoloid slant
>Varicose veins, hernia or uterine or rectal prolapse
>Mitral valve prolapse

Requirement for Diagnosis
>Any one of the following:
>- 2 major criteria
>- 1 major plus 2 minor criteria
>- 4 minor criteria
>- 2 minor criteria & unequivocally affected first degree relative in family history

Tissue Healing Process

Following an injury, the body's soft tissue structures undertake a natural healing process through specific stages of healing. These stages involve the replacement of destroyed tissue with living tissue (Figure 2.2).

WOUND HEALING

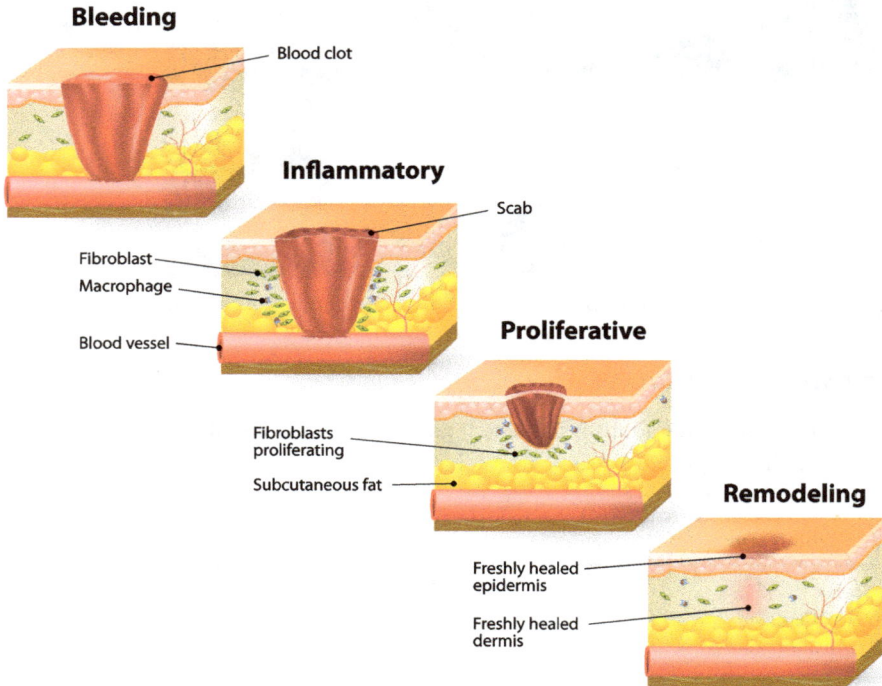

Bleeding

Blood clot

Inflammatory

Scab

Fibroblast

Macrophage

Blood vessel

Proliferative

Fibroblasts
proliferating

Subcutaneous fat

Remodeling

Freshly healed
epidermis

Freshly healed
dermis

FIGURE 2.2 The wound healing process.

Fractures

A bone fracture is where the continuity of the bone is broken. A fracture can range from a thin crack to a complete break. Bone can fracture transversely, linearly, in several places or into many pieces (Figure 2.3). Most fractures happen when a bone is impacted by more force or pressure than it can support.

Types of Bone Fractures

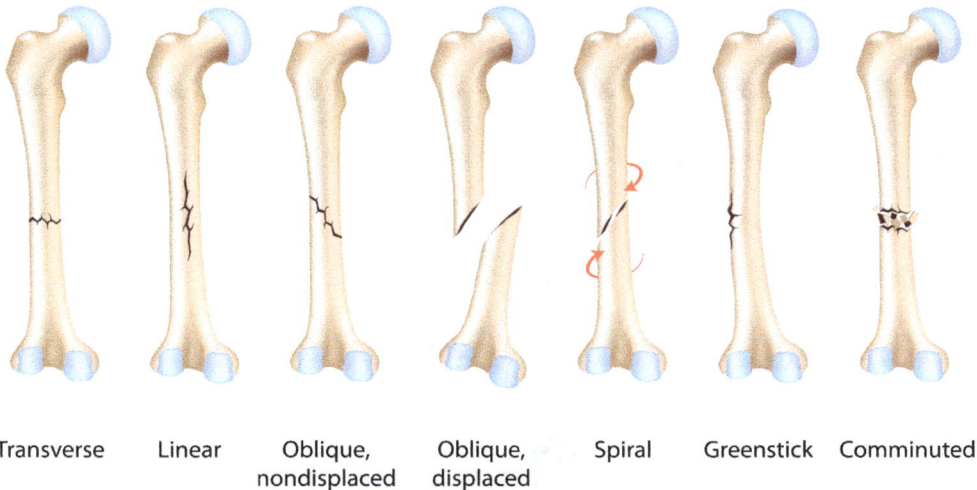

| Transverse | Linear | Oblique, nondisplaced | Oblique, displaced | Spiral | Greenstick | Comminuted |

FIGURE 2.3 Different types of bone fractures.

Grades of Ligament Injury

Ligaments attach bone to bone, although strong and rigid, strains and sudden forces can cause them to rupture and tear. Damage is caused when the fibres become torn and the severity depends on the extent to which the ligament has torn.

- Grade I – mild ligament tear
- Grade II – moderate incomplete ligament tear
- Grade III – complete ligament tear

Muscle Strains

A muscle strain is an injury to a muscle either in the muscle belly or at the musculotendinous junction. Minor strains may only overstretch these tissues, while more severe injuries may involve partial or complete tears of these tissues. Muscle strains can be graded (Table 2.6).

TABLE 2.6 Muscle strain grading criteria

Grade	Description
1	Mild strain, no loss of function. <5% muscle involved, focal oedema or haemorrhage
2	Moderate strain, reduced strength of musculotendinous unit, >5% muscle involvement, mild fibre rupture, increased oedema/haemorrhage
3	Severe strain, significant fascial tearing, significant to complete muscle fibre disruption, significant oedema/haemorrhage

Other classifications are widely used in the industry. It is good to know your sports and the common classification system used for it, for example the Munich consensus statement (2012) and the British Athletics Muscle Injury Classification (2014) [2–3].

Neurodynamic and Neuro-integrity Tests

A neurodynamic assessment evaluates the length and mobility of the nervous system. They are performed by the sport rehabilitator placing progressively more tension on the component of the nervous system that is being tested. Testing is divided into upper limb and lower limb.

Lower Limb Neurodynamic Tests

Straight Leg Raise– SLR (Sciatic nerve) (Figure 2.4)

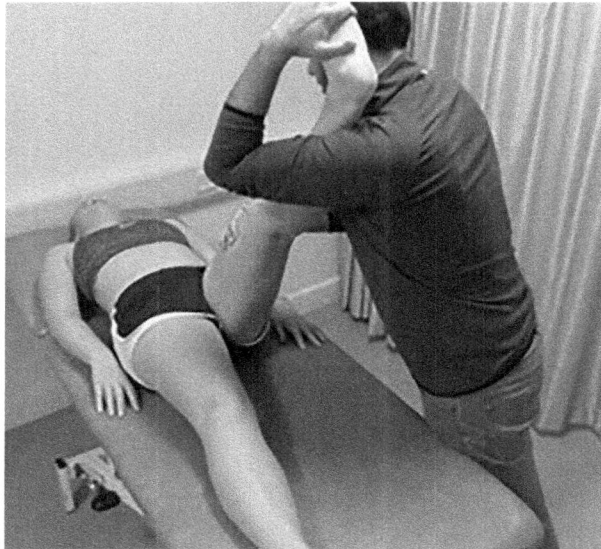

FIGURE 2.4   Straight leg raise test.

- Client is supine
- IR of hip, then flexion, with knee extended
- Ankle dorsiflexion (tibial nerve)
- Ankle plantarflexion and foot inversion (common peroneal nerve)
- Hip adduction (sciatic nerve)
- Increasing hip IR (sciatic nerve)
- Passive neck flexion (spinal cord, meninges and sciatic nerve)

Prone Knee Bend – PKB (Femoral nerve tension test) (Figure 2.5)

- Client side lying on unaffected side
- Unaffected side: client grasping tibia in full hip flexion
- Affected side: passive hip extension with full knee flexion
- Thoracic and cervical spine flexed
- Cervical extension is the desensitising test

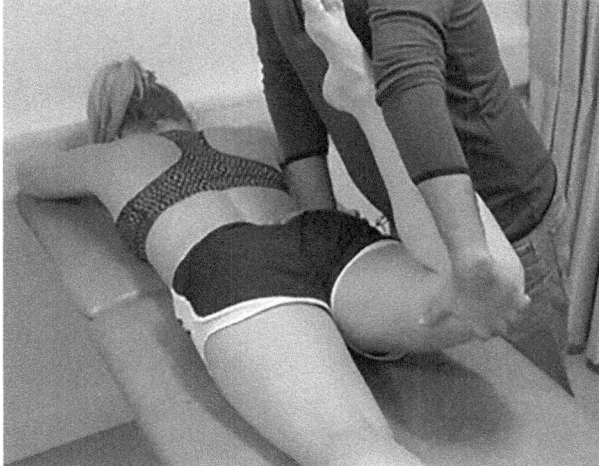

FIGURE 2.5 Prone knee bend test.

Slump Test (Figure 2.6)

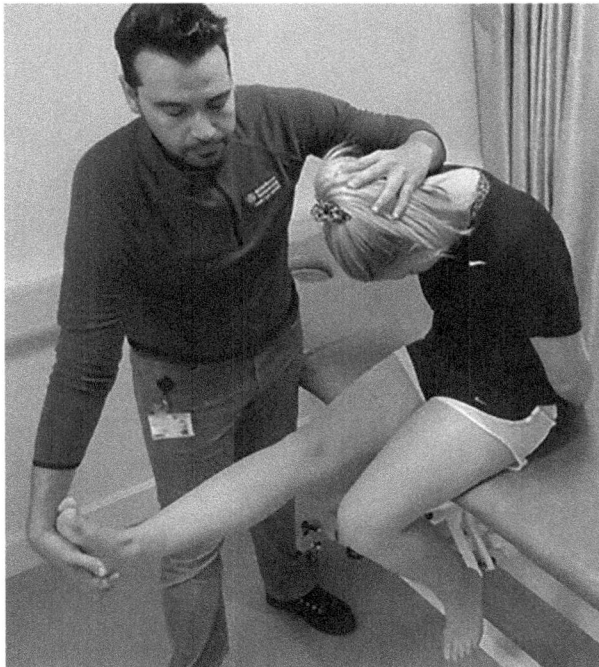

FIGURE 2.6 Slump test.

- Client's hands behind back
- Thoracic flexion
- Cervical flexion (chin to chest)
- Extend one knee

- Dorsiflex foot of extended knee
- Cervical extension to desensitise
- Extend other leg with cervical flexion

Upper Limb Neurodynamic Tests

Upper Limb Tension Test 1 (ULTT1) – Median nerve bias (Figure 2.7)

- Shoulder girdle depression
- Shoulder abduction
- Shoulder external rotation
- Forearm supination
- Wrist and finger extension
- Elbow extension
- Cervical spine side flexion (contralateral side)

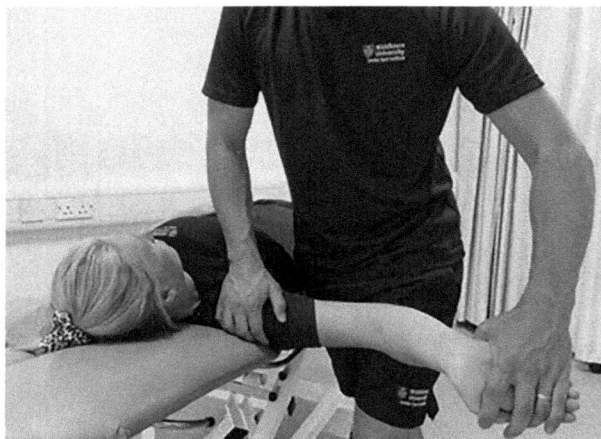

FIGURE 2.7 ULTT1.

Upper Limb Tension Test 2a (ULTT2a) – Median nerve bias (Figure 2.8)

- Shoulder girdle depression
- Elbow extension
- Lateral rotation of the whole arm (thumb pointing downwards)
- Wrist, finger and thumb extension

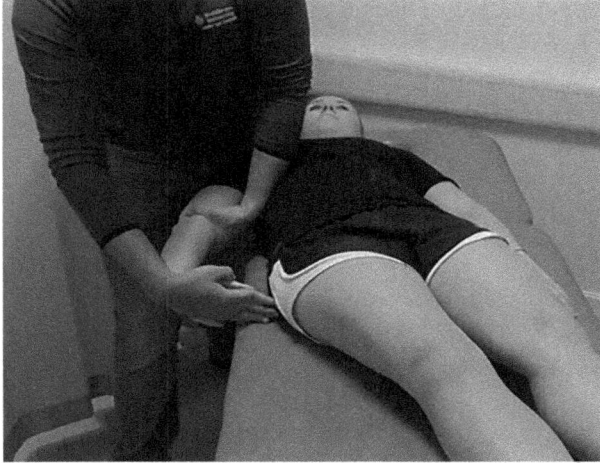

FIGURE 2.8   ULTT2a.

Upper Limb Tension Test 2b (ULTT2b) – Radial nerve bias (Figure 2.9)

*   Shoulder girdle depression
*   Elbow extension
*   Medial rotation of the whole arm (thumb downwards)
*   Wrist, finger and thumb flexion
*   Shoulder abduction
*   Cervical spine contralateral side flexion

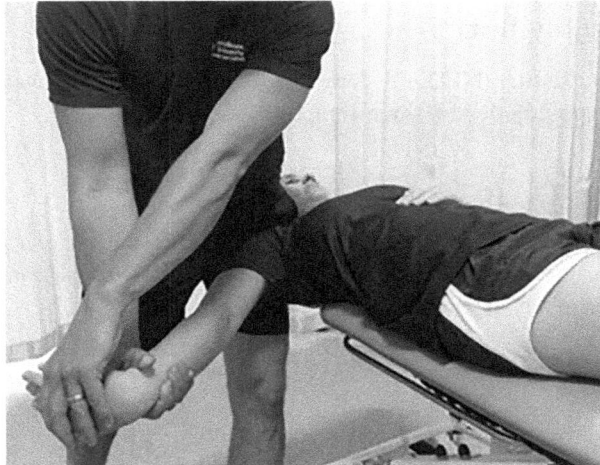

FIGURE 2.9   ULTT2b.

Upper Limb Tension Test 3 (ULTT3) – Ulna nerve bias (Figure 2.10)

- Shoulder girdle depression
- Shoulder abduction
- Shoulder external rotation
- Wrist pronation
- Wrist and finger extension
- Elbow flexion
- Shoulder abduction
- Cervical spine contralateral side flexion

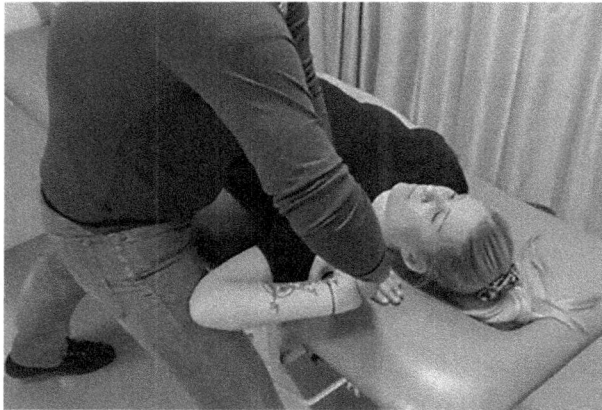

FIGURE 2.10   ULTT3.

Neurological Integrity Tests

Neurological Integrity Testing (NIT) – A complete test is dermatomes, myotomes and reflexes – the test is not complete without ALL three components.

Dermatomes

A *dermatome* is the area of the skin that is mainly supplied by branches of a single spinal sensory nerve root. These spinal sensory nerves enter the nerve root at the spinal cord and their branches reach to the body's periphery (Figure 2.11).

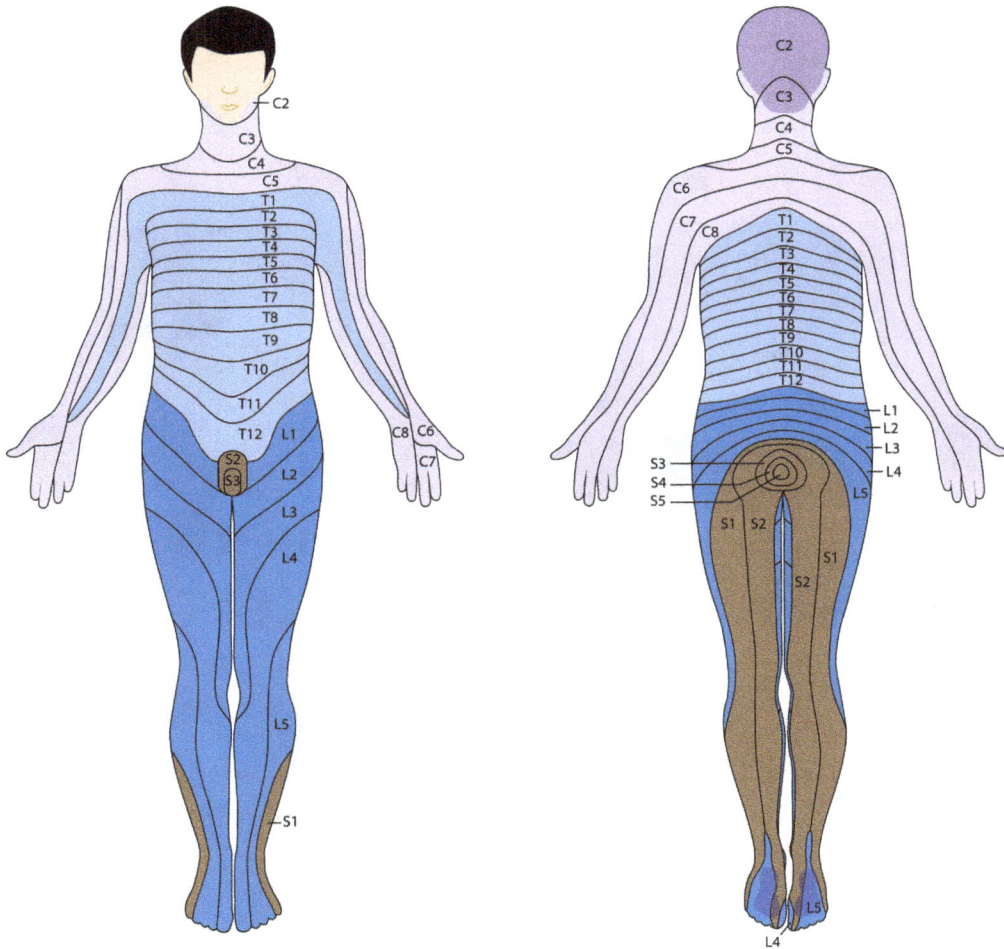

FIGURE 2.11 Dermatomal areas within the body.

Myotomes

A *myotome* is a group of muscles innervated by a single spinal nerve root.

C1 – Neck flexion
C2 – Neck extension
C3 – Neck side flexion
C4 – Shoulder elevation
C5 – Shoulder abduction
C6 – Elbow flexion wrist extension
C7 – Elbow extension
C8 – Finger flexion
T1 – Finger abduction
L2 – Hip flexion
L3 – Knee extension
L4 – Ankle dorsiflexion
L5 – Great toe extension
S1 – Ankle plantarflexion

Reflexes

Reflexes are involuntary contractions of a muscle caused by the activation of muscle spindles. They are elicited by a sudden stretch of the muscle induced by a quick hammer strike on the muscle tendon (Figure 2.12). Note the reflex response and compare both sides. Decreased reflexes can be a sign of spinal nerve and peripheral nerve damage (Table 2.7).

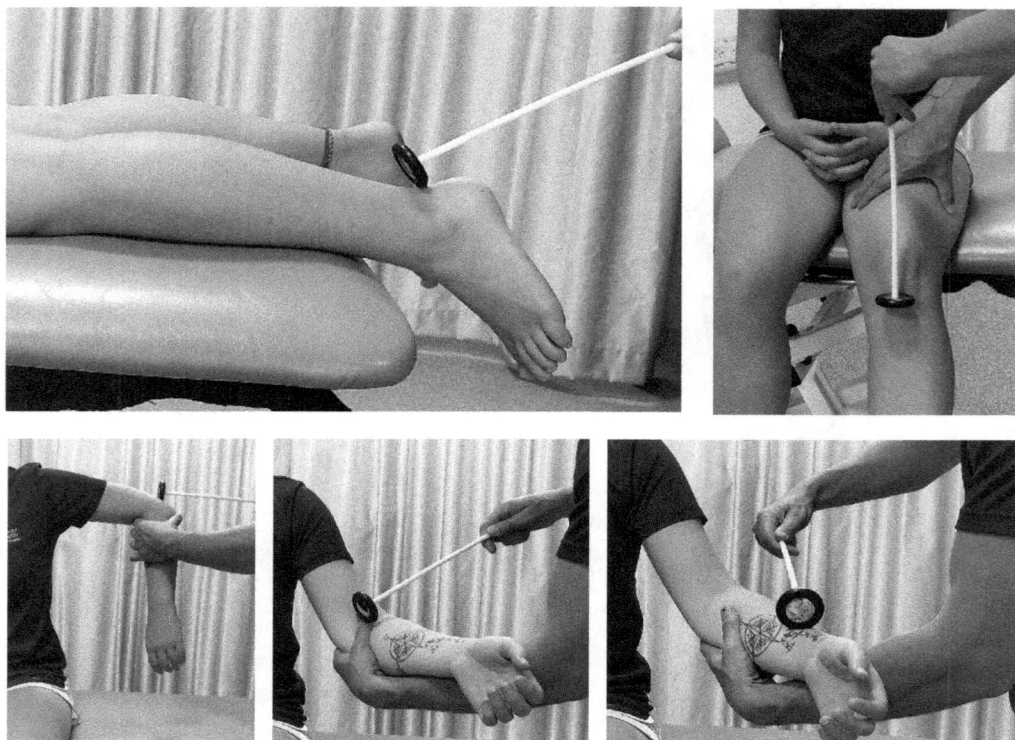

FIGURE 2.12   Reflex testing for the upper lower limb and upper limb.

TABLE 2.7 Reflex response grading criteria

Grading	Client response
Absent	No muscle contraction or tendon response
Diminished	A small or slow reaction
Normal	A muscle contraction happens or a tendon response
Increased	Quick or exaggerated response
Brisk with or without clonus	A rhythmic muscle spasm indicative of an upper motor lesion

Postural Assessment Screening

Postural assessment looks at a client's static posture to identify if there are any imbalances or abnormalities that could be causing pain, discomfort or attributing to injury. It is important to assess the client in the anterior (Figure 2.13), lateral (Figure 2.14) and posterior view (Figure 2.15).

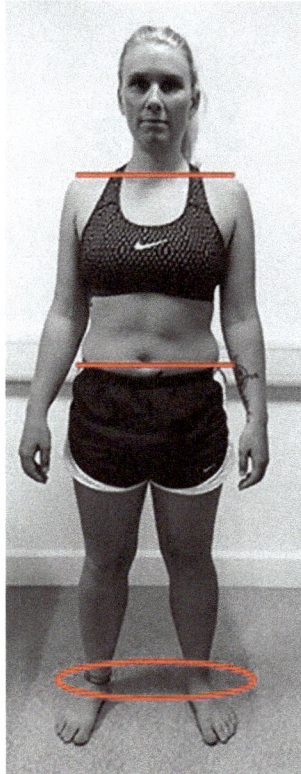

FIGURE 2.13   Postural assessment, anterior view.

Anterior View

Foot and Ankles:
Straight and parallel, not flattened or externally rotated?

Knees:
In line with toes, not add or abducted?

LPHC:
Pelvis level with both ASIS level?

Shoulders:
Level and not elevated or rounded?
Position of arms – internally or externally rotated?

Head:
Neutral not tilted or rotated?

Lateral View

Foot and Ankles:
Heels flat on floor?

Knees:
Neutral knees or are they hyperextended or flexed?

LPHC:
Neutral pelvic position, anterior or posterior pelvic tilt?

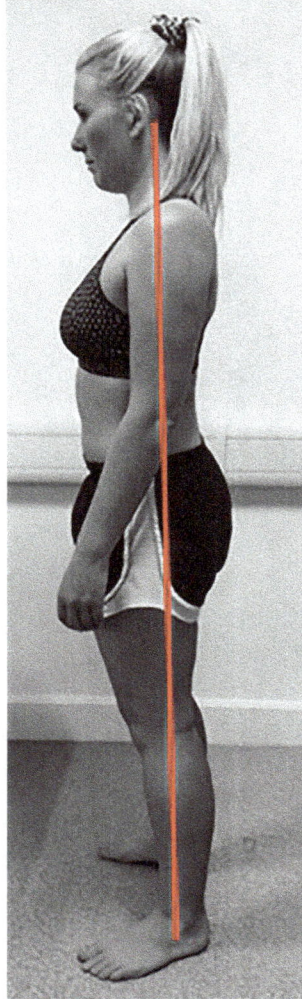

FIGURE 2.14 Postural assessment, lateral view.

Mid Thoracic and Shoulders:
Neutral thoracic curve or kyphotic?
Rounded shoulders?
Head:
Neutral position, forward head posture?

Posterior View

Foot and Ankles:
Heels are neutral, no protonation of ankle, external rotation of feet?

Knees:
Knee creases equal?
Knee valgus/varus?

LPHC:
PSIS level, iliac crest level?

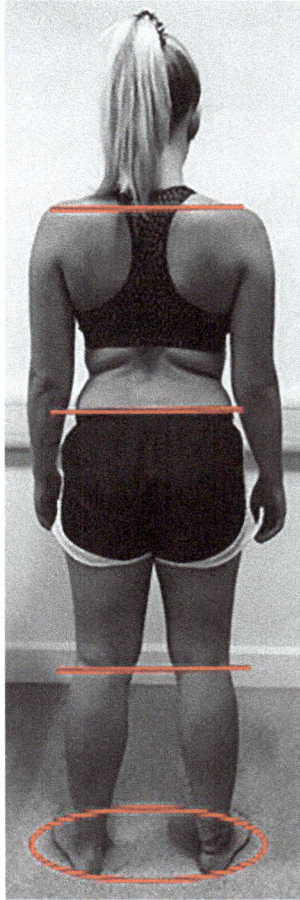

FIGURE 2.15   Postural assessment, posterior view.

Shoulders:
Scapula level, not winging?
Shoulders level not elevated?
Arm rotation angle?

Head:
Ears level?

Common Postures

Posture can be defined as the way the body is supported during muscular activity or as a result of coordinated muscle activity working towards maintaining stability. Poor posture can be recognised as a faulty relationship of the various parts of the body which produces increased strain on the supporting structures and in which there is less efficient balance of the body over its base of support [1].

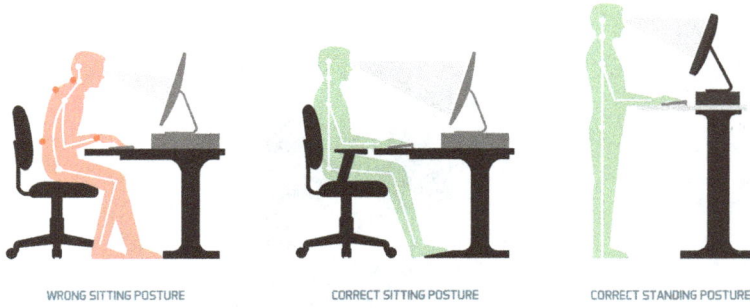

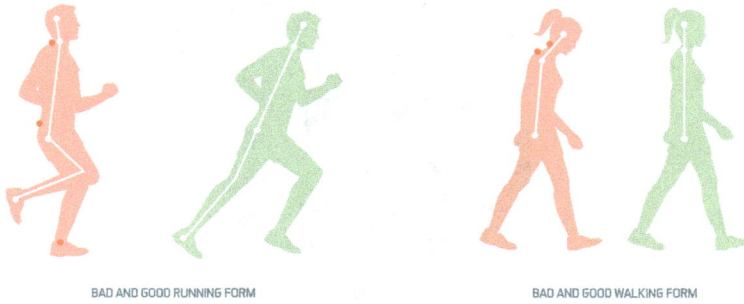

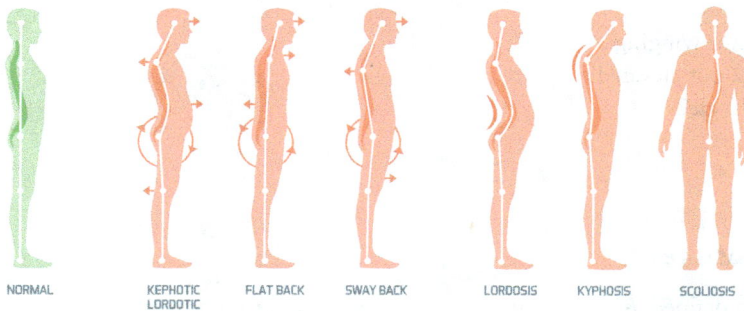

FIGURE 2.16 Common body postures with normal activities of daily living.

Functional Assessment Tests

Functional assessment tests can be a way of identifying movement restrictions or asymmetry. These assessments involve the rating of movement quality from the sports rehabilitator and/or using measurements (Figure 2.17, 2.18, 2.19).

Overhead Squat (OHS)

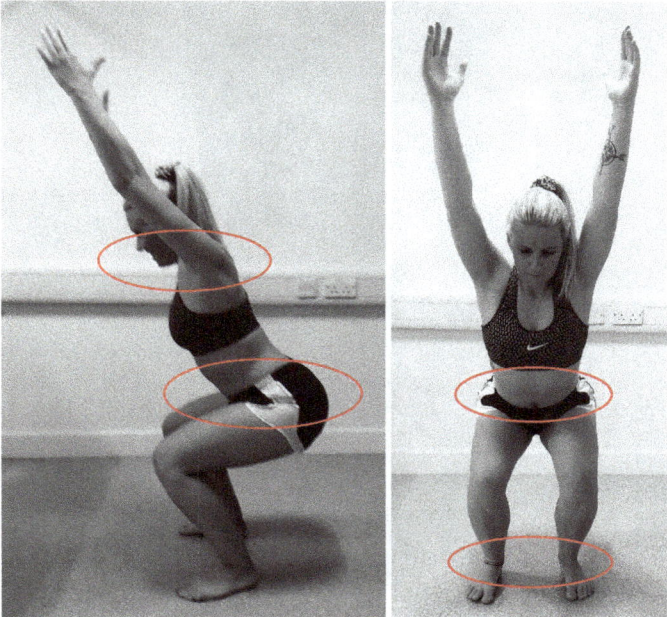

FIGURE 2.17   Overhead squat test.

Single Leg Squat (SLS)

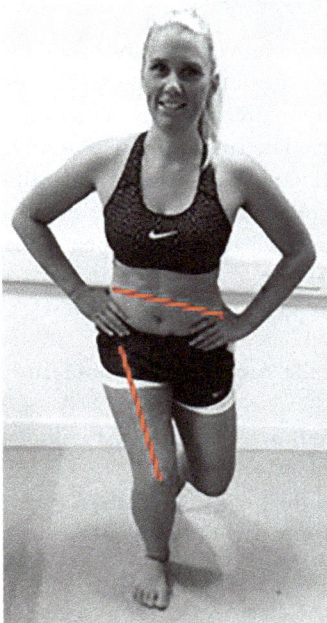

FIGURE 2.18   Single leg squat test.

Knee-to-wall (KTW)

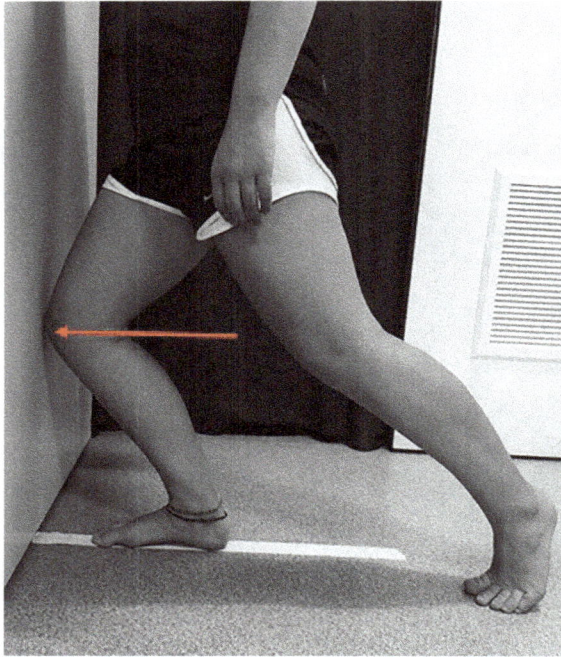

FIGURE 2.19 The knee-to-wall test.

Functional Movement Score (FMS)

This screening tool is used to identify movement limitations and limb asymmetries by examining a combination of strength, balance, flexibility, range of motion and coordination during seven selected movement patterns. The sports rehabilitator scores the athletes from 0 to 3 as they complete each of the seven movements. The sum of these scores is then used to identify the athletes' functional movement. The FMS (Figure 2.20) has been identified as having high intra–rater reliability (ICC = 0.98). In addition, researchers have identified that athletes with lower FMS scores were more likely to incur injury in comparison with their higher-scoring counterparts [4, 5].

FMS Scoring

3 = the individual can perform the movement without any compensations according to the established criteria.

2 = the individual can perform the movement but must utilise poor mechanics and compensatory patterns to accomplish the movement.

1 = the individual cannot perform the movement pattern even with compensations.

0 = the individual has pain during any part of the movement.

The Functional Movement Screen

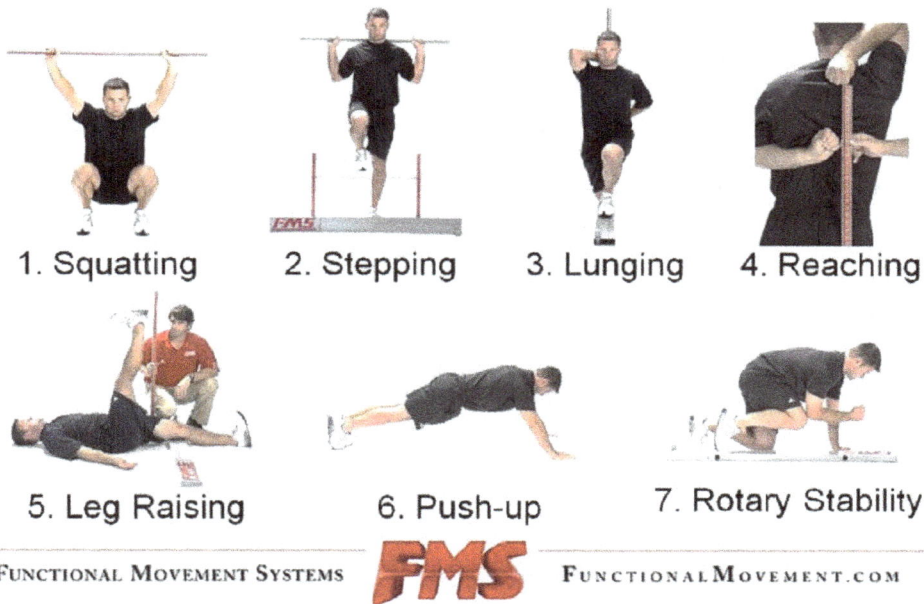

1. Squatting 2. Stepping 3. Lunging 4. Reaching

5. Leg Raising 6. Push-up 7. Rotary Stability

FUNCTIONAL MOVEMENT SYSTEMS **FMS** FUNCTIONALMOVEMENT.COM

FIGURE 2.20 The seven testing stages of the FMS.

Client Initial Assessment

The initial assessment (subjective and objective) is an essential part of the client examination as it helps determine the severity, irritability and nature (SIN) of the patient's condition. Thorough questioning is paramount in guiding the sports rehabilitator to form a diagnosis, treatment plan and an injury prognosis.

Initial Assessment Structure

Client's name, DOB and **page numbers** should be clear on all pages.

Subjective Assessment

Present Condition (PC) – what the client has come to see you about.
History of Present Condition (HPC) – what, when and how.
Past Medical History (PMH) – previous accidents, injuries, surgeries.
Drug History (DH) – medications.
Social History (SH) – occupation and recreational activities.
Aggs and Eases – what aggravates and what eases the current symptoms.
24-Hour Pattern – is the pain worse in the morning, afternoon, evening?
Special Questions

- T.H.R.E.A.D.S (**T**hyroid, **H**eart, **R**heumatoid **A**rthritis, **E**pilepsy, **A**sthma, **D**iabetes, **S**teroids)
- Red Flags – Signs of serious pathology. (Cauda equina syndrome, fracture, tumour, unremitting night pain, sudden weight loss of 4.5 kg over 3 months, bladder and bowel incontinence, previous history of cancer, saddle anaesthesia.)

  If you suspect any red flags the patient must seek urgent medical attention and it is better to send the patient to AandE rather than risk any permanent, life-changing pathology.
- Yellow Flags – Psychosocial concerns. (Unhelpful beliefs about pain: indication of injury as uncontrollable or likely to worsen. Expectations of poor treatment outcome, delayed return to work. Distress not meeting criteria for diagnosis of mental disorder. Worry, fears, anxiety.)

Objective Assessment (O.P.P.ROM.S.S.)

Observation – how a client moves naturally.
Posture – how the client stands/sits. Symmetry or asymmetries.
Palpation – pain, heat, bony landmarks, muscles, ligaments.
Range of Movement – active and passive.
Strength – MMT and BT.
Special Tests – orthopaedic and functional tests.
Clinical Impression – diagnosis.
Treatment (Rx) – manual therapy, electrotherapies, modalities, exercise prescription.
Re-Test – identify if treatment has been successful.
Plan – next follow-up appointment.

Follow-up Assessment (SOAP notes)

Subjective – changes since last appointment?
Objective – re-assess previous clinical findings.
Assessment – (special tests, clinical impression, treatment (Rx), Re-test post Rx.
Plan – next follow-up appointment.

References

1. Pollock, N., James, S. L., Lee, J. C., & Chakraverty, R. (2014). British athletics muscle injury classification: a new grading system. *British journal of sports medicine, 48*(18), 1347–1351. https://doi.org/10.1136/bjsports-2013-093302
2. Kendall, F., McCreary, E. K., Provance, P. G., McIntyre Rodgers, M., & Romani, W. A. (2005). *Muscle testing and function with posture and pain* (5th ed.). Philadelphia, PA: Lippincott Williams & Wilkins.
3. Kiesel, K., Plisky, P. J., & Voight, M. L. (2007). Can serious injury in professional football be predicted by a preseason functional movement screen? *North American journal of sports physical therapy, 2*(3), 147–158.
4. Loffing, F., Hagemann, N., Strauss, B., & MacMahon, C. (2016). *Laterality in sports theories and applications*. London: Elsevier.
5. Mueller-Wohlfahrt, H., Haensel, L., Mithoefer, K., Ekstrand, J., English, B., McNally, S., Orchard, J., Niek van Dijk, C., Kerkhoffs, G. M., Schamash, P., Blottner, D., Swaerd, L., Goedhart, E., & Ueblacker, P. (2013). Terminology and classification of muscle injuries in sport: The Munich consensus statement. *British journal of sports medicine, 47*, 342–350.

3

SPORTS INJURIES

Sarah Budd

Tendinopathy

Tendinopathy is a generic term that describes tendon disruption or tendon disorders [1]. This can then be further broken down and includes both tendinitis and tendinosis. Tendinitis is the inflammation of a tendon whilst tendinosis often refers to the degeneration of a tendon, they both generally fall into the category of chronic tendon injury. Chronic tendon problems can occur in all tendons; however, some locations tend to be predisposed to injury such as the patella tendon, Achilles, groin and rotator cuff tendons.

Mechanism of Injury: The pathogenesis of tendinopathy is extremely complex and multifactorial [2], there is still more developments to be made in the research behind it to help us have a better understanding. Chronic tendon injury is associated with abnormal load, either a sudden increase in load or an acute change in the frequency, volume or intensity of load [3–6]. Overload has been known in cause microtrauma and degeneration, causing a failure in the healing process of the tendon [2]. Along with this, factors such as genes, gender, age, high BMI and biomechanics, in particular at the foot in relation to Achilles tendinopathy, have also been known to contribute [5–7].

Symptoms: Some cases of tendinopathy can be asymptomatic; however, one of the most common symptoms is pain. The pain often changes depending on the stage of tendon dysfunction, but often the more load placed on a tendon, the more pain experienced [6]. Early in the phases of tendinopathy pain often comes on during loading but improves with as the activity goes on and subsides completely as load ceases. Tendon pain is often localised and does not spread, episodes of early morning stiffness in the Achilles tendon are also common [6]. Weakness in the affected limb is often present along with tenderness on palpation of the affected tendon. Swelling is not always and rarely present, however; thickening or crepitus may be present in peri-tendon pathology [6].

Treatment: Treatment of tendinopathy depends on several factors: location, gender, age, level of activity, to name a few. It is important to review the latest research related to the specific case when putting together a treatment plan [8]. Treatments are broken down into those that aim to treat pain and then those that aim to change pathology.

Exercise-based interventions have been discussed as being one of the most effective treatment methods for mid-portion Achilles tendinopathy [4]. Eccentric exercise, including heavy eccentric calf training, otherwise known as the Alfredson protocol, has been shown to have positive effects as a treatment for mid-portion Achilles tendinopathy; however, it is less effective in other locations [4]. Exercise programmes that focus on load-based rehabilitation should be progressive [7],load management is important and getting consistent and progressive load works well for tendon pathology, complete rest should be avoided. Isometric contractions of the quadriceps have been known to induce analgesia in patella tendinopathy and are often prescribed as part of a warmup for athletes suffering from tendon pain [7]. If biomechanics are a contributing factor, then this should also be considered as part of the exercise-based rehabilitation programme [6].

Shockwave therapy has been shown to offer positive effects on pain when combined with exercise therapy [9]. Along with this, acupuncture has also been shown to have positive results when combined with both shockwave and exercise therapy [9]. However, those modalities that focus on pain reduction often do not have long-term effects and it is common for recurrence to occur [6].

Both platelet-rich plasma (PRP) and autologous blood injections have had some positive results in helping to reduce symptoms and improve healing on the degenerative tendon; there has also been some research to suggest this, in addition to other modalities such as acupuncture/needling, have had positive results [10].

It is important to understand that there still needs to be further research to develop a 'gold standard approach' to the management of tendinopathy, and that due to its complexity, this may not exist and a 'one size fits all' is not the right approach.

The Lower Leg and Ankle Complex

Lateral Ankle Sprain

Mechanism of Injury: The most common mechanism of a lateral ankle sprain (LAS) is inversion, with or without planta flexion of the ankle [11]. LAS can occur due to contact or non-contact; non-contact is often due to landing from a jump and the ankle 'rolls' and contact is often due to a direct contact such as a tackle (Figure 3.1).

Symptoms: Symptom severity will depend on the grade and severity of the injury and damage. Swelling will often be present; however, this is not a good indicator of the injury severity. Along with this there may be bruising located around the antero-lateral area of the ankle and foot. The anterior talo-fibular ligament is often the most injured ligament and will be tender on palpation. Pain will occur when moving the ankle into inversion and plantar flexion, and deficits in range of movement may also be seen in dorsi flexion and eversion. There will often be weakness of surrounding muscles and, depending on severity, patients may find it difficult to bear weight fully due to pain.

Treatment: In an acute LAS, PEACE & LOVE should be followed. Immediate care should follow PEACE and then following this management should follow LOVE. This will optimise recovery and allow for sufficient soft tissue healing [12]. Early management has been shown to modulate the healing process and speed up return to sport for athletes and daily living for general population [13].Functional support has been presented as being useful in allowing patients to load damaged tissues in a protective manner [14]. This has been shown to have better outcomes in comparison to immobilisation.

Joint mobilisations have also been shown to have positive effects on pain following an acute lateral ankle sprain. A range of techniques including the Mulligan Concept and talocrural joint mobilisations have been shown to improve outcome post-acute LAS [15–16].

Rehabilitation is an important part of the management of LAS. It is not uncommon for patients to suffer chronic ankle instability and recurrent sprains [13–14]. Exercise-based rehabilitation

Ankle Sprains

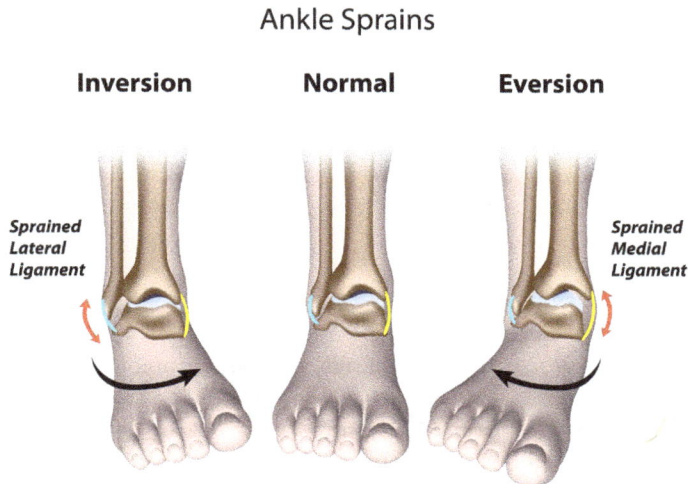

FIGURE 3.1 The mechanism of a medial and lateral ankle sprain.

should start early and involve resuming normal range of movement, some form of proprioceptive and neuromuscular training/exercises. Strength work should focus on the intrinsic foot muscles and calf complex. Recent research has identified that the use of an impairment-based rehabilitation model may be useful when treating LAS and potentially reduce the risk of chronic ankle instability [17]. Surgical intervention for LAS, despite good clinical outcomes, is not the preferred method for treatment of acute or chronic injuries. Conservative management is seen to be more suitable due to reduced exposure of invasive treatment and the potential for risk of complications [18].

Compartment Syndrome

Mechanism of Injury: compartment syndrome is a condition where pressure increases within a space within the limb and then compromises the neurovascular supply. Compartment syndrome can be categorised into chronic or acute; acute compartment syndrome is caused by acute trauma such as a fracture, bleeding or swelling in a non-elastic muscle compartment normally from direct impact. Chronic compartment syndrome (CCS) is common in young athletes and occurs during strenuous exercise due to the increase in pressure, and from recurrent muscle cramping and tightness [19–20].

Symptoms: The most common symptoms are pain and swelling which are made worse by exercise and physical activity. The pain is normally out of character for the injury/clinical situation. In CCS pain normally starts early on in exercise and eases once activity has stopped. Pain is aggravated with stretching the affected muscle group, for example with anterior compartment syndrome the pain would increase with plantar flexion [11, 21]. The area will be warm to touch and sometimes the skin glossy. Looking out for the five Ps of an impending compartment syndrome are important: Pain, Paraesthesia, Pallor, Pulselessness and Paralysis. Paralysis of the muscles in the affected compartments and the loss of an arterial pulse are recognised as being late signs of compartment syndrome. In CCS pain normally starts early on in exercise and eases once activity has stopped [21].

Treatment: Immediate recognition and referral for treatment are extremely important with compartment syndrome if it is left untreated muscle ischemia and tissue necrosis can occur.

It is recommended that all compartments should be decompressed surgically [22], conservative management if often unsuccessful. Aggravating exercise should be stopped, and normal physical activity will need to be modified depending on pain, it is important to know that pain often resume without surgical intervention. Post-surgery early mobilisation is important and gradual return to exercise can be considered including the use of hydrotherapy and stationary cycling [21].

Calf Strain

Mechanism: Calf muscle injuries are common in a multitude of sports, with acute episodes common in sports that involve high volumes of running load, high-speed running, jumping, acceleration and deceleration and change of direction [23–25]. Calf injuries tend to have a longer average time of return to sport and tend to have increased reoccurrence rates [26].

The gastrocnemius has previously been found to be the higher risk calf muscle due to it crossing two joints and the higher density of type two muscle fibres [27], in comparison to the soleus and plantaris muscles of the calf complex. However, recent evidence has shown soleus injuries to be more prevalent in certain sports such as Australian League Football and Tennis [25, 28]. The soleus is made up or largely type 1 fibres and therefore is more subject to gradual onset injuries, but also makes up a larger physiological cross-sectional area.

There is strong evidence to suggest that previous calf injury increases the risk of further calf injury and some evidence to suggest that other lower limb injury to both soft tissue and joint can predispose patients to a calf muscle injury [25–26]. Age has also been shown to demonstrate strong evidence of increasing risk of calf injury; this is due to a loss of skeletal muscle tissue quality and function [26–29].

Research has shown that calf muscle injuries are more likely to occur during high competition times such as the end of the competitive season in football [30].

Symptoms: For injuries involving the soleus muscle symptoms include calf tightness/stiffness, pain that worsens over a longer period of time and aggravated by walking and jogging [1, 27]. Gastrocnemius strains tend to present with pain in the medial belly or the musculotendon junction, whereas the soleus more lateral [1]. One factor for differentiating between the two muscles is isolating either muscle, by adding or removing full knee extension; this is due to the anatomical location and the soleus not crossing the knee joint like the gastrocnemius [1].

Treatment: Acute calf strains can be treated using either POLICE or PEACE and LOVE protocols in the early phase but then exercise-based rehabilitation should commence, especially in the active population. Early onset of rehabilitation has been shown to reduce return-to-sport time in athletes by around three weeks without any increased risk of injury [29]. Leaving the muscle to de-condition or atrophy can be detrimental. It is important to note, however, that injuries involving connective tissue will take longer to heal and have a higher risk of failure [28].

Rehabilitation should consist of progressive isometric loading to aid with pain modulation and tendon stiffness and then the addition of concentric and eccentric exercise to increase rate of force development and fascicle length. Later-stage rehabilitation should focus on increasing explosiveness; the use of Olympic lifting has been shown to be useful for this, high-speed running, jumping/landing and plyometric-focused exercises. Blood-flow restriction training has also shown positive effects in increasing muscle size with low load on the muscle. Rehabilitation should be continued for at least six months post injury; a focus on heavy calf work either isometric or eccentric is key.

Plantar Fascia Pain

Plantar fascia pain has been given several different terms over the years, which often causes a lack of understanding on the pathology – terminology such as plantar fasciitis, plantar heel pain, runners' heel, plantar fasciopathy, to name a few. It has been recognised that a consensus on appropriate nomenclature for the condition should be considered [31].

Mechanism: Plantar heel pain is an overuse condition that is one of the most common causes of foot pain [3, 32] and is very common in long-distance runners. It involves the plantar aponeurosis of the foot and repetitive strain causing micro tears to the tissues, which in turn induce a healing response[32–34]. Previously thought to be an inflammatory condition, it is now thought to be a degenerative condition [32]. Plantar fascia pain is known to be multifactorial with a number of associated causative factors. In the athletic population it is often caused by overload or sudden changes in load, like tendon pathology.

A pes planus, flattened foot with forefoot pronation or pes cavus, high-arched foot are often found in symptomatic patients and are seen to be contributing factors [35–38]. A reduction in dorsiflexion at the 1st MTPJ is also considered risk factors along with a reduction in the strength of the intrinsic foot muscles that support the longitudinal arch [38]. In the non-athletic population high body mass index is one of the most common risk factors [35–36], probably due to the higher biomechanical load [37]. Along with this, an increased age has also been found to be an associated risk [35].

Symptoms: Patients often describe medial plantar heel pain when weight bearing; pain and stiffness are often worse first thing in the morning that often eases with rest [32]. There may be pain on palpation of the plantar fascia, more so medial side, and pain with passive dorsiflexion and big toe flexion (known as the windlass test). Foot muscle and ankle dorsiflexor weakness are often associated symptoms [39, 40].

Treatment: There are a number of treatments that have been used for plantar fascia pain. High numbers of patients are treated conservatively, without the need for surgery [32]; however, treatment can take anything up to 12 months [40]. Treatments include managing the acute symptoms such as pain; this can be done via the use of modalities like cryotherapy, non-steroidal anti-inflammatories (NSAIDs) and rest [32]. It is important to understand that the use of NSAIDs should be used for pain relief and not to counteract the pathophysiology, due to inflammation not always being present [40]. The use of corticosteroids has long been discussed; however, most research suggests that the long-term effects come with associated risk [32]. There is also evidence to suggest the use of extracorporeal shock wave therapy (ESWT) has demonstrated good or excellent improvements in pain [40]. However, research is still not conclusive (Figure 3.2).

Treatment should also comprise trying to treat contributing factors, for example the use of orthotics to correct foot biomechanics and alignment, corrective exercise to help improve strength of the lumbopelvic hip complex and intrinsic foot strength along with stretching of the calf complex and foot muscles. Superior effects have been seen when the use of orthotics combined with stretching have been used [32, 40].

When trying to treat the source of symptoms, there has been a large amount of research that has gone into finding optimal treatments. In the more recent research, exercise-based rehabilitation consisting of eccentric and heavy, slow resistance training have been highlighted to be a superior method of treatment [39, 41]. Alternative treatments such as platelet-rich plasma have also been considered to promote healing of the injured tissues [40].

Surgical intervention can be considered if after 6–12 months conservative management has failed; treatment would then include a complete or partial plantar fasciotomy [32, 42].

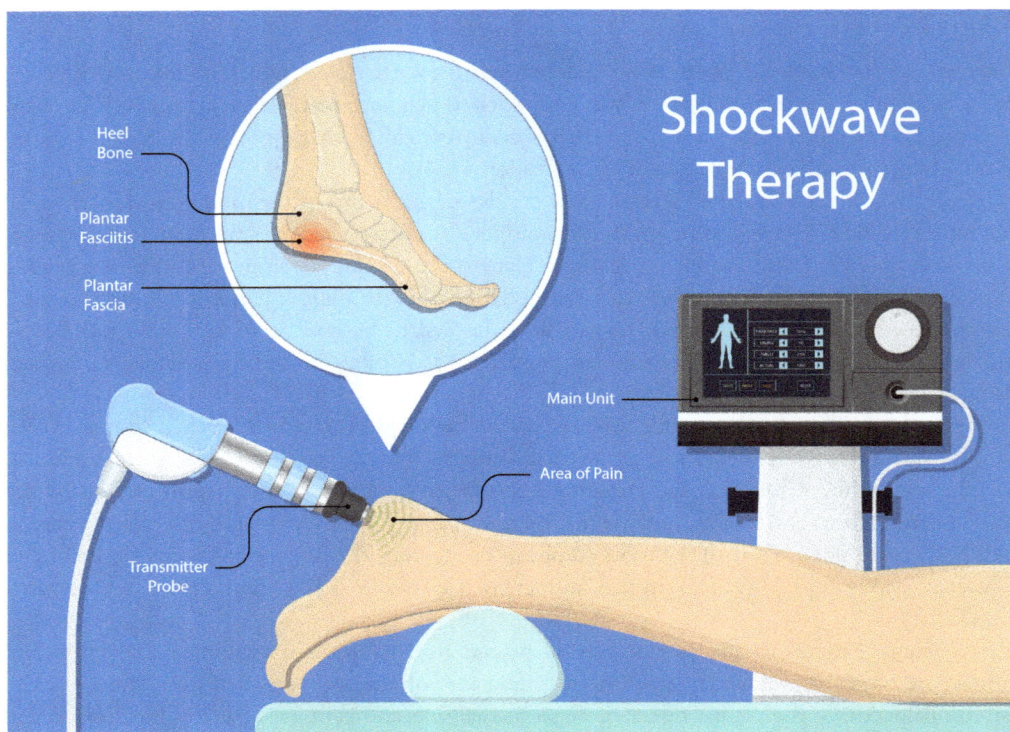

FIGURE 3.2 Shockwave therapy.

The Knee

Anterior Cruciate Ligament Rupture

Mechanism: Over 70% of anterior cruciate ligament (ACL) injuries (Figure 3.3) are non-contact [43–44]. The most common movements occurring, in the lead up to an ACL injury are known to be; a cut and plant movement, sudden change of direction or speed, abrupt deceleration moments, pivoting, twisting and landing with less than 30° of knee flexion [45–46]. Most non-contact ACL injuries occur with the valgus collapse movement; this includes combined movements of knee flexion + internal rotation + anterior tibial displacement + knee valgus [47].

Females are four to five times more likely to suffer an ACL compared to males [1]. There are many other risk factors involved with an ACL injury; these include ligament laxity, bone morphology, training load and techniques, reduced strength and limb symmetry and poor neuromuscular control [48–49].

Contact ACL injuries are often due to direct impact to the injured knee, either directly to the lateral side of the knee or lower limb, with a forced valgus collapse and hyperextension [46].

Symptoms: Symptoms of an ACL rupture may include an audible pop or crack at the time of the injury, swelling of the knee joint that comes on immediately or soon after the injury. Feelings of instability, more so if a more complex injury involved other structures in the knee, restricted movements with the inability to fully extend the knee. On assessment of the knee joint there will be increased anterior tibial translation with little end feel and often rotational instability.

Treatment: ACL ruptures can be managed either with surgical reconstruction (ACLR) or conservative management. The chosen treatment method will be dependent on several factors; the

TEAR OF THE ANTERIOR CRUCIATE LIGAMENT (ACL)
MEDIAL VIEW OF THE KNEE

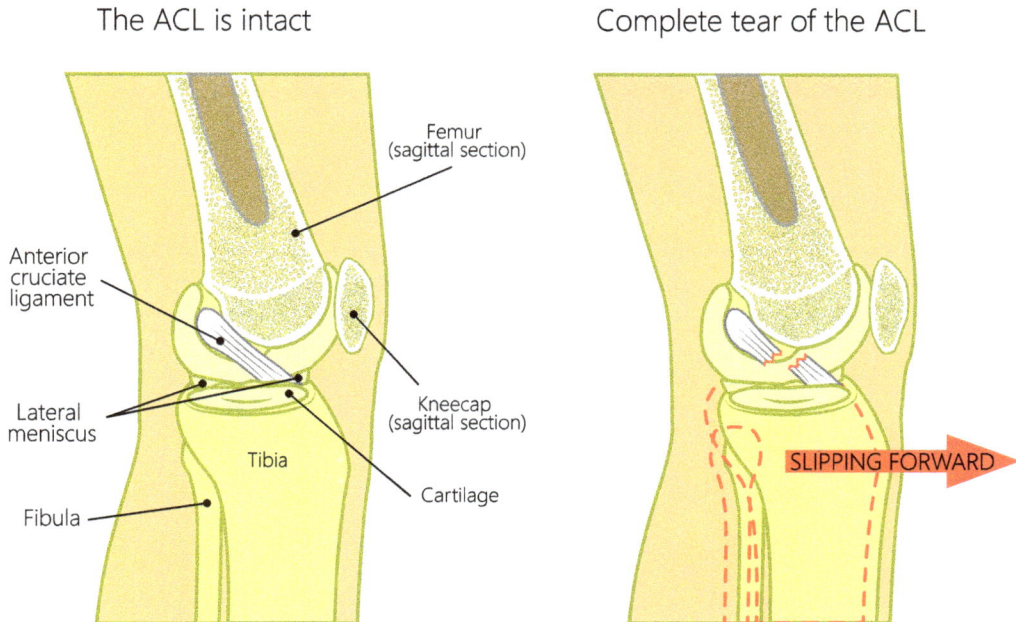

FIGURE 3.3 Tear of the anterior cruciate ligament.

patient's age, activity level, adherence to rehabilitation, surgical risk factors, functional disability and whether the injury is isolated to the ACL only. It is often recommended that athletes involved in sports that require large amounts of cutting, pivoting and sudden deceleration to undergo surgical reconstruction; however, there is no single predictor as to whether an ACL-deficient patient should undergo surgical reconstruction or exercise-based rehabilitation only [50].

Surgical reconstructions include the use of either an allograft or autograft. Autografts are normally taken from the patient's ipsilateral or contralateral hamstring tendon or patella tendon. A lateral tenodesis is sometimes utilised to control anterolateral laxity and contribute to decreased pivot shift [51].

What is known is that whether surgical reconstruction is the choice of treatment or not, a criteria-based rehabilitation programme should be completed to enable a safe return to sport and reduction in the risk of re-injury. Time alone should not be the deciding factor in returning to play, no matter the route of treatment.

In the acute stage post injury or post surgery, it is important to focus on regaining full range of motion at the knee, in particular, knee extension, and by reducing muscle atrophy as much as possible by the introduction of early movement, weight bearing and gait re-education where possible and the introduction of muscle activation exercises in safe ranges of movement. Cryotherapy can be used early on to reduce swelling and pain.

When considering a rehabilitation plan for an ACL injury many things should be included; focus on restoring lower limb strength is extremely important, with a good symmetry of the quadricep and hamstring muscles, in relation to both interlimb and intralimb. Good neuromuscular control is essential in reducing the risk of re-injury, along with efficient mechanics of the trunk, hip and knee [48]. Once appropriate lower limb strength and neuromuscular control have been gained, progression to return to running, and sports specific tasks should also be undertaken [52]. It is important that during the rehabilitation period, clear goals are set for the athlete to progress from one stage to another and specific outcome measures are met to determine readiness to return to sport [52].

It is recommended any athlete that has suffered an ACL injury complete an injury prevention programme long-term to reduce their risk of injury [48, 51, 53].

Posterior Cruciate Ligament

Mechanism: Posterior cruciate ligament (PCL) sprains are much less common than other ligaments in the knee such as the ACL or medical collateral ligament due to its great strength [54–55]. The mechanism of injury is often a direct blow on the anterior aspect of a flexed knee causing excessive force posterior [54, 56] (Figure 3.4). In sport this type of injury would normally occur from a direct blow such as a tackle in football. In the general population, PCL injuries are known as the 'dashboard injury' and occur from a high velocity trauma such as a road traffic accident [54, 56]. Other mechanisms include falling onto a flexed knee with a plantar flexed foot or a sudden hyper-extension of the knee [54].

Symptoms: Symptoms often include pain in the posterior aspect of the knee and the posterolateral corner/joint line may be tender on palpation. Depending on the severity of the injury the fibular head may also present with tenderness. There may be some swelling, but not as much as the swelling people experience after an ACL sprain, due to the extra synovial anatomy. Often there is some mild bruising around the popliteal fossa of the knee.

On movement, pain is often increased with knee flexion past 90 degrees and therefore aggravated by deep squatting or kneeling [55]. There may be some weakness of the quadriceps and hamstring muscles. On other functional assessment patients may complain of a feeling of instability, pain on sprinting and deceleration in particular [57].

There are several orthopaedic tests that may present symptoms of pain and laxity but visually the posterior sag test often demonstrates obvious loss of control of tibia translation if a complete rupture has occurred [56].

It is uncommon for patients to hear a 'pop' sound commonly heard when suffering a high-grade sprain of the ACL, and it is sometimes the case that patients are able to continue the activity they were taking part in during the injury. PCL injuries are often seen less acutely as patients can develop symptoms over time in isolated injuries [55].

Treatment: With isolated PCL injuries, especially low-grade injuries, there is research to support the use of conservative management focusing on an extensive exercise-based rehabilitation; good return to sport rates and successful outcomes have been identified [54–56, 58]. For more complex injuries, if numerous structures are damaged and there is significant instability in the knee then surgery may be considered [54]. There is still inconclusive evidence as to the management of high-grade PCL injuries; factors that should be considered are level of activity, symptomatic laxity and functional competency of the knee [55].

Bracing: immobilisation of the knee and protected weight-bearing post PCL injury is common, keeping the knee in full extension for 2–4 weeks before commencing rehabilitation [55–56, 58].

Exercise-based rehabilitation should focus on regaining knee range of movement early, avoiding hyperextension [59], normalising gait and building strength. It is important to limit large degrees of flexion and hamstring activity to ensure limited posterior translation forces in the earlier stages of rehab [54–55, 59]. Rehabilitation should focus on both open and close kinetic chain exercises; these exercises are particularly indicated early on due to the co-contraction of the hamstrings and quadriceps, reducing patellofemoral stress and tibia translation [54]. Stability should be a key focus of rehabilitation, along with control of the lumbopelvic hip complex.

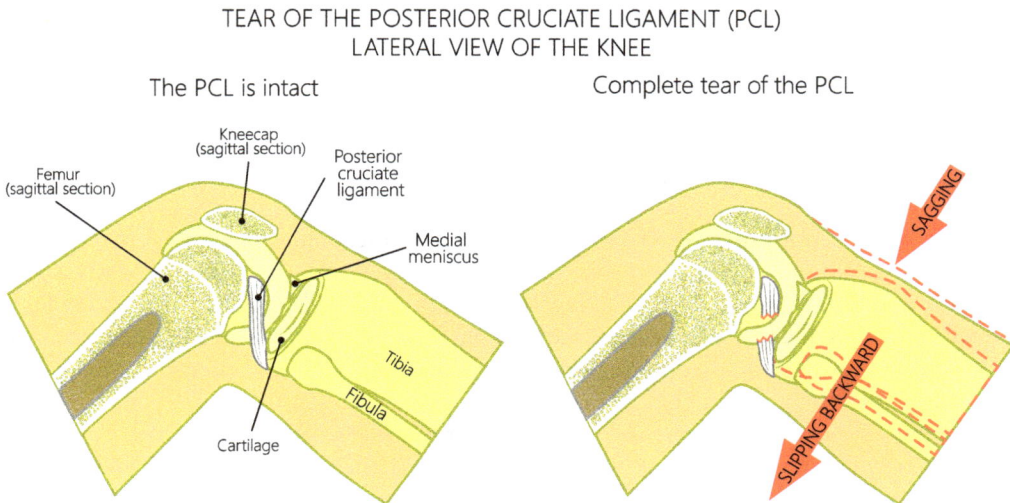

FIGURE 3.4   Tear of the posterior cruciate ligament.

Medial Collateral Ligament Sprain

Mechanism of Injury: Medial collateral ligament (MCL) injuries are extremely common injuries that occur in athletes and the sporting population. They often occur due to contact to the lateral aspect of the knee or leg whilst the foot is planted into the ground, applying valgus force, and stressing the MCL. MCL injuries can also occur in non-contact scenarios; these often occur due to rotational or valgus stress that occurs in sudden change of direction, landing, or deceleration. It is not uncommon for the MCL to become injured alongside other structures such as the ACL, posterior cruciate ligament, and menisci [60–61].

Symptoms: Symptoms will differ depending on the grading and severity of the injury; however, it is not uncommon to hear an audible 'pop' at the time of injury followed by immediate swelling or swelling within 48 hours of the injury. Pain is also often present around the medial knee joint and over the MCL itself. Laxity will likely be present; if present when performing a stress test in 30 degrees of flexion but not zero degrees, this indicates an isolated MCL injury, whereas both indicate a multi-ligament injury [60–61].

Treatment: Treatment often depends on the severity of the damage to the MCL and if it is an isolated MCL or multi-ligament injury. Most non-complex, isolated MCL injuries can be treated conservatively without the need for surgical intervention [62]. When treating with exercise-based rehabilitation the focus should be to encourage early restoration of a normal range of motion, to reduce muscle atrophy, in particular the quadriceps group and then progress to increasing lower limb stability and strength of the knee and hip complex. The use of a non-restrictive hinged knee brace has been shown to help reduce the risk of valgus instability early on; however it is important, particularly in grade I and II injuries, that range of motion is not compromised [60, 62]. Early weight bearing should be encouraged and restricted only by symptoms; restoration of normal gait should be of importance in the rehab programme. Manual therapy might be used to compliment exercise-based rehab including patella mobilisations, soft tissue therapy and friction massage.

If conservative management fails and persistent instability is present then surgical intervention may be required; this is also the case with multi-ligament and more complex cases [60].

Osgood-Schlatter Disease

Mechanism of Injury: Osgood-Schlatter Disease (OSD) is found commonly in adolescents and is described as painful lumps or inflammation of the tibial tuberosity (TT) [63]. It is a traction apophysitis at the level of the tibial tubercle [64] which is the attachment point for the patella tendon. This has been known to be vulnerable to high stress before maturation [64]. OCD often occurs due to repetitive strain from the quadriceps musculotendinous junction at the TT [65], therefore sports that involve repetitive knee extension are risk factors [66]. However, OSD is seen to appear in children and adolescents during a growth period and is not always linked to sports activity [66]; this is due to bones and cartilage growing much quicker than muscles and tendons in an adolescent growth spurt, thus putting strong force on to the site of the insertion of the patella tendon [67].

Symptoms: Pain is often a symptom, which increases during or after sports activity, especially intense activity, but in the early stages will reduce at rest [67]. Particularly, pain tends to be present in activities such as walking up and down stairs, jumping, squatting and direct contact or kneeling. Pain can also be elicited on resisted knee extension from bent knee position; however, resisted straight leg raise is normally painless. OSD can also be characterised by enlarged TT [68–69], along with tenderness on palpation of the TT [56]. Tightness or reduced range of movement in the quadriceps muscles can also be present [70].

There are three stages of OSD described by Wall [66]:

- Stage I: Pain withdraws after physical activity within 24 hours.
- Stage II: Pain occurs only after physical activity, but it is not restricting and does not disappear within 24 hours.
- Stage III: Permanent pain which limits not only physical but also everyday activities.

Treatment: Previous research has stated that most cases of OSD resolve within 12–18 months without long-lasting implications; however, this is now being questioned and current evidence suggests that it is too optimistic to expect this type of condition to not cause lasting problems [64]. Implications may affect athletes' strength and function years after symptom resolution [71–72] and this therefore puts them at risk of further musculoskeletal problems [64].

The Hip

Hamstring Strain

Mechanism of Injury: Hamstring strain injuries (HSI) are an extremely common injury to occurs in athletes of a variety of sports, generally sports that include high-speed running, kicking, and sudden deceleration. Sprinting or high-speed running (HSR) seem to be the most widely reported events leading up to a HSI [73–74]. When looking into the biomechanics of a HSI, they often

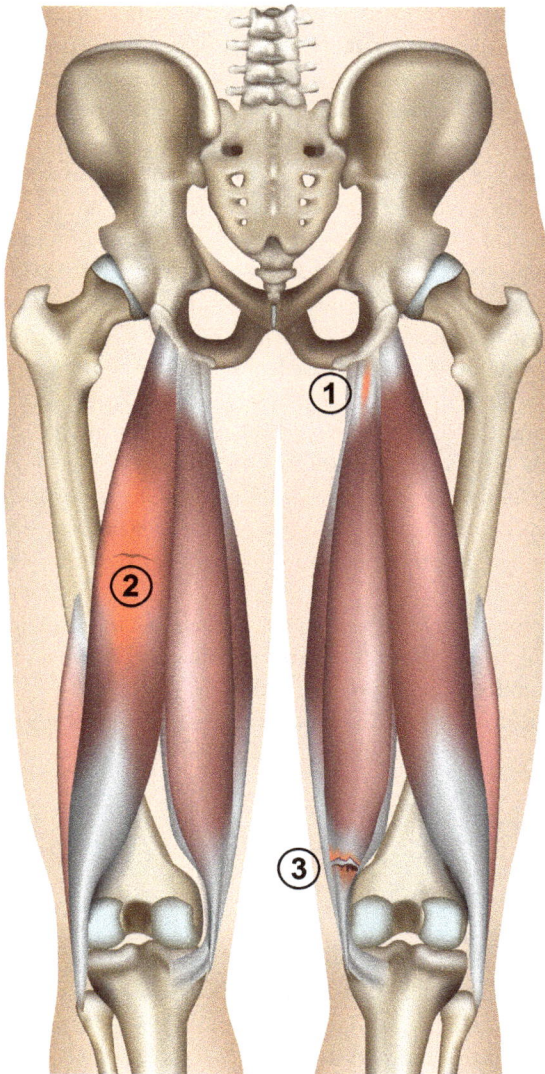

Types of hamstring injuries

1.Grade
Less than 5% of muscle tendons
cracked
(Slight swelling, slight
Pain, no loss of strength)

2.Grade
Multiple fibers injured
(Significant loss of power with strong
Pain)

3.Grade
Tearing of muscles / tendons
(Loss of muscle function with
Hematoma)

FIGURE 3.5   The types of hamstring injuries with associated symptoms.

occur during eccentric contraction, and they have been commonly seen in the late swing phase of sprinting [75]. However, it has been reported that a peak knee flexion movement and a peak hip extension movement post foot strike have been common mechanisms leading up to a hamstring injury [75]. Both stretching and kicking have also been reported as mechanisms of HIS [74]. Other risk factors for a HSI include lack of muscle fascicle length, an imbalance or loss of strength in the hamstring muscle particularly eccentric knee flexion strength [76] and increased neural tension [75]. Non-modifiable risk factors include age, and previous HSI [75–76].

Symptoms: HSI is often present with a sudden onset of pain in the posterior thigh; the severity of the pain will vary depending on the patient and injury severity. Sometimes a popping or tearing sensation can be felt or heard. Bruising may occur up to several days post injury as well as potential swelling and warmth of the injury site. Pain on sitting can also be present in the event of a proximal musculotendinous junction (MTJ) strain or avulsion injury at the ischial tuberosity (Figure 3.5). Other symptoms include a loss in hamstring flexibility or hip and knee range of movement, loss of hamstring strength with pain on contraction. Neural tightness may also be present during a slump test.

Treatment: As with most soft tissue injuries, treatment protocols are dependent on the severity and complexity of the injury. There have, however, been many studies focusing on ways to manage hamstring injuries through exercise-based rehabilitation and ongoing injury prevention programmes (IPP) due to high re-injury rates. Loading should be initiated early after an HSI but in a safe manner to reduce the risk of further injury. Tissue healing should be considered, and POLICE has been well presented as a protocol to follow [77].

Rehabilitation should start gradually and be progressive. Isometric hamstring exercises can begin early on in rehabilitation, progressing to concentric and then eccentric exercises. Rehabilitation and IPP should then focus on eccentric strength training using both unilateral and bilateral exercises, the Nordic hamstring exercise has been heavily researched and found to be beneficial, along with exercises such as the Askling Glider and diver [78], stiff leg deadlifts and rear foot elevated split squats. Strength should focus in improving muscle imbalance and general hamstring strength. Other areas to focus on are general conditioning, exposure to high-speed running and plyometrics [74].

Core strengthening exercise and proprioception have been shown to influence HSI due to the change in pelvic position and hamstring length and therefor gait during running. These should therefore be factors considered when programming a rehabilitation plan [79].

In severe HSI that involve the MTJ, due to the high incidence of re-injury rates surgical opinion may be taken, especially with athletes involved in sports associated with plenty of high-speed running and sprinting moments.

Spinal Conditions

Low Back Pain

Mechanism of Injury: Non-specific low back (LBP) pain refers to pain in the lumbar spine with the absence of a specific pathology. LBP is often multifactorial, and many risk factors are associated. It is characterised by a range of biophysical, psychological, and social dimensions [80]. Females are much more likely to report LBP compared to males and prevalence has been shown to increase with certain lifestyle factors such as obesity, poor general health, a history of depression, smoking, and low levels of activity [81–82]. There has also been some correlation between LBP and biomechanical factors such as poor posture and a lack of kinetic chain function. Weaknesses in core musculature and hip mobility have been shown to affect LBP [82].

Symptoms: One of the most common symptoms is general pain in the low back region. This can vary from moderate to severe, often first thing in the morning or towards the end of the day [80]. Pain is not associated with a specific pathology and red flags are not present. Patients often present with fear avoidance of movement and generally have high anxiety around their LBP. An acute episode can last up to around 6 weeks with more chronic episodes lasting for 12 weeks or more [83]. If the LBP is due to a postural dysfunction this may be present on observation or joint assessment, with lack of mobility and strength being present; there might also be evidence of a pelvic tilt, normally anterior and a leg length discrepancy.

Treatment: Treatment of low back should focus on being educational and follow a biopsycho-social model. NICE guidelines do not recommend imaging unless the clinician believes the results would change the management plan; NICEguidelines suggest encouraging the patient to be active and follow an exercise-based rehabilitation programme; it is important to consider the patients' needs and capabilities when prescribing a programme and choosing the type of exercise. Offering Pilates-based exercise, hydrotherapy and a day-to-day increase in activity levels are appropriate starting points.

Education should be reassuring and aim to help the patient understand the complaint, its cause and likely outcome, as well as explaining that no medical treatment or required for many patients [81].

Spondylolisthesis

Mechanism of Injury: Spondylolisthesis is the term for a spectrum of disease that is characterised by the movement (often anterior) of one vertebral body in relation to another. Spondylolisthesis can be congenital, acquired or due to idiopathic causes. The most common part of the spine for this to occur is in the lumbar portion, but it can also occur in the cervical spine, and normally only due to trauma; in the thoracic spine.

According to the Wiltse Classification [85] there are five types of spondylolisthesis:

I   Dysplastic
II   Isthmic
IIA   With disruption due to stress fracture
IIB   Elongation of the part without disruption
IIC   Acute fracture through pars
III   Degenerative
IV   Traumatic
V   Pathologic

Degenerative types commonly occur in female adults compared to male adults; obesity is known to increase the risk of this type. Isthmic types are more common in adolescents and young adults and tend to be more common in males than females, but other possible risks include microtrauma from sports such as gymnastics and activities involving repeated lumbar extension. Traumatic spondylolisthesis manifests after pars interarticularis fractures and commonly occurs after trauma. Pathologic types occur due to bone or connective tissue disorders including infection. Dysplastic types mostly occur in children, predominantly females.

Symptoms: Symptoms for patients often include localised pain in the region/spinal segment of the pathology, often aggravated by flexion and extension of the affected spinal segment. Pain is normally eased by lying in a supine position. Pain is not uncommonly radicular caused by narrowing of the nerve foramina, with pain sometimes presenting in the gluteal muscles, numbness and or weakness in the legs [84, 86].

Treatment: For low-grade injuries spondylolisthesis is often treated conservatively including treatments such as exercise-based rehabilitation, and NSAIDs, and initially a period of rest avoiding movements and activities that exacerbate symptoms [87]. Exercise-based rehabilitation should focus on spinal and hip mobility including increasing hamstring length if reduced, along with strength-based exercises with a key focus on the core. Core exercises should include some dynamic work to focus on balance and stability along with strength [88]. Hydrotherapy has been shown to improve symptoms such as pain whilst also providing a safe yet suitable environment to develop mobility, stability, strength, and cardiovascular fitness. It has also been more recently discussed that when treating a patient with spondylolisthesis a biopsychosocial model and approach should be used to reduce disability and thoughts [89].

If conservative management fails, which is roughly in around 10–15% of younger patients [87], then surgical treatment may be required. Surgical options vary from decompression, and fusion; however, there is no gold standard approach at current.

Spondylolysis

Mechanism of Injury: Spondylolysis is a bony defect in the pars interarticularis or isthmus of the vertebrae; it can occur unilaterally or bilaterally and is most common in the lumbar spine but can affect all spinal segments. Spondylolysis risk in increased in several populations; athletic, specific ethnic groups and age; generally, it develops younger and is more common in males. Wynne-Davies also found that there may be a genetic factor involved [90].

The condition is common in athletes such as gymnasts, weightlifters, wrestlers, and swimmers due to mechanical stress and repetitive load on the spine, and it is not often caused by one traumatic event [91]. The mechanical stress is heightened during movements such as extension and rotation and is most affected at L5 due to repeated hyperextension [91–93].

Symptoms: It is not uncommon for spondylolysis to be asymptomatic; it is often found incidentally on imaging. When a patient is symptomatic, symptoms may consist of low back pain often aggravated by extension. Pain is often intense and comes on after activity; pain can also radiate into the gluteal region and thigh if the condition is present in the lumbar region [93].

Treatment: Most symptomatic cases can be treated conservatively with the focus to be on reducing levels of pain and facilitating the healing process of the vertebrae. Exacerbating activities should be restricted whilst undertaking an exercise-based rehabilitation programme. Rehabilitation should focus on core strengthening and restoration of mobility including hamstring length if restricted, and then returning the patient to the pre-injury level of activity. In cases, bracing is often considered alongside conservative treatment [93–95]. If conservative management fails and persistent pain occurs, or development of neurological deficit, then surgical intervention may be needed [95].

Shoulder

Rotator Cuff Tear

Mechanism if injury: The rotator cuff muscle group are one of the most injured muscle groups and can often have long-term effects on active daily living [11, 96]. Acute rotator cuff injuries often happen due to fall on an outstretched hand (FOOSH) and direct fall onto the shoulder itself. This can cause compression and inflammation to occur or traction and tearing of the muscle. It is uncommon for an acute traumatic tear to occur at the rotator cuff; full thickness tears are more often due to chronic, repetitive trauma or underlying condition [11]. Those that are at higher risk, however, are athletes involved in overhead and contact sports such as swimming, rugby and tennis [96–97]. Other factors that are involved in rotator cuff tears are impingement, age and pathology just as thyroid disorder, diabetes and inflammatory conditions.

Symptoms: The specific anatomy and location of the tear will influence symptoms and dysfunction; however, symptoms that may be present are reduced shoulder range of motion, weakness and atrophy of the involved muscle, pain with overhead activity, night pain and pain when lying on the affected shoulder and painful arc sign [11, 98–99]. When palpating the shoulder, tenderness may be present anteriorly; palpating the cuff tendon defect is an effective method to diagnosing full-thickness rotator cuff tears. This can be done by palpating anterior to the acromion with the shoulder in extension and will disappear with the shoulder in flexion [99]. Due to weakness in the rotator cuff muscles it is not uncommon to see scapular dyskinesia and altered scapulohumeral rhythm during shoulder movement [99].

Treatment: Treatment methods vary from conservative to surgical interventions; often chronic and degenerative tears are treated conservatively whereas more recent research suggests that an acute/traumatic tear should be treated with surgical intervention [100]. It is not uncommon for conservative management to fail, and to decrease pain, surgical intervention to repair the tear has been known to be successful; however, further research is needed to form a definitive decision on the management.

Research has shown conservative treatment to be successful, with good clinical outcomes after 12 months [101]. When focusing on conservative treatment, exercise-based rehabilitation should focus on regaining normal shoulder movement including restoring good scapular control and position. If scapular dyskinesia is present this should be targeted [99]. Exercises focused on unloading the rotator cuff are helpful in the early stages with the progression active assisted and then isometric strength work of the rotator cuff and scapular stabilisers [101]. Progressive rehabilitation building strength and the power and plyometric activity are important for athletes returning to sport.

If conservative management fails, then surgical intervention should be considered.

Shoulder Impingement

Mechanism of Injury: Impingement at the shoulder occurs when there is a decrease in the sub acromial space, the area in which the supraspinatus and sub acromial bursa pass through [11]. Impingement can be due to several factors, primarily because of compression of the rotator cuff tendons due to structural changes that narrow the subacromial space. The shape of the acromion process can play a role in primary impingements. Secondly, due to underlying conditions such as glenohumeral joint instability causing increased humeral head translation and poor scapulothoracic movement and internal causing repetitive contact of the posterior greater tuberosity and posterior-superior glenoid rim [102–103]. Muscle imbalance has been known to play a big role in SI, causing poor posture and a lack of shoulder range of movement, all of which are known contributing factors (Figure 3.6).

Symptoms: Symptoms of shoulder impingement include persistent pain without a specific mechanism of injury or trauma [54], patients often report a 'painful arc'; moving the arm between 70 and 120 degrees of abduction, and overhead movements that affect daily living. Pain is also often present when lying on the affected side, particularly at night with sleep sometimes being affected. Pain is not often localised but described anatomically around the anterior glenohumeral area.

Treatment: Treatment should focus on decreasing pain and regaining good function of the shoulder joints including the scapular. Conservative management should always be the first choice with surgery only being considered if the patient does not improve with conservative management [104].

In the acute phase treatments that can be considered are avoidance of aggravating activities or movements, and the progressing onto an exercise-based rehabilitation programme. Research has shown good outcomes from exercise-based rehabilitation, especially when combined with other

Normal Shoulder

Clavicle

Supraspinatus
Muscle

Acromion

Bursa

Humerus

Supraspinatus
Tendon
(Rotator Cuff)

Coracoid
Process

Glenoid

Scapula

Shoulder Impingement

Arthritic
Deformation

Trapped
Tendon
and Bursa

Inflammation

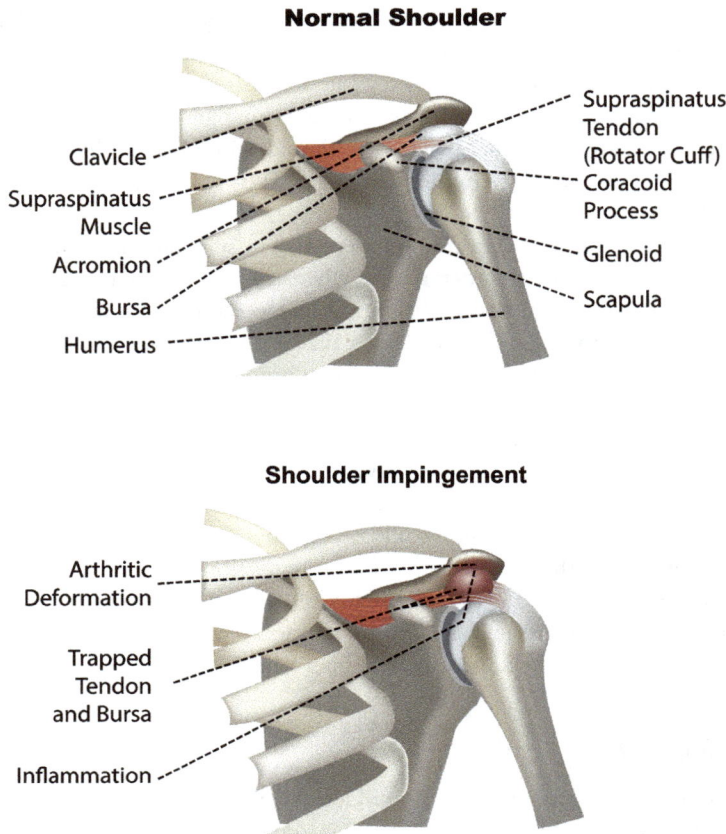

FIGURE 3.6 A normal vs impinged shoulder joint.

modalities such as manual therapy, kinesio taping and acupuncture therapy [105]. Rehabilitation should focus on restoring optimal range of movement at the shoulder, increasing both rotator cuff and scapular strength along with proprioception and stabilisation at both the shoulder and scapular [103]. A mix of both open and closed kinetic chain exercises have been shown to beneficial with focus on working on all planes of movements including scapular setting exercises [106–107].

Acromioclavicular Joint Sprain

Mechanism of Injury: The acromioclavicular joint (ACJ) is the most commonly sprained joint in the shoulder complex [11]. Injuries to the ACJ and associated ligaments normally occur from a fall onto an outstretched hard (FOOSH) [59] but most commonly from direct contact onto the point of the shoulder, often with the arm in adduction. This forces the acromion caudally into the clavicle [11].

Symptoms: Symptoms often depend on the severity/grading of the injury but AJC sprains are usually associated with symptoms such as localised pain and point tenderness, effusion and swelling over the joint, pain with shoulder movement particularly abduction past 120 degrees [54]. Elevation of the clavicle may also be present if second- or third-degree injury.

ACJ Classification, adapted from Rockwood's Classification 1996 [54]:

I: A sprain of the AC joint capsule accompanied by localised pain and tenderness on palpation and movement, especially horizontal flexion.

II: Complete rupture of the AC ligament complex, accompanied by a sprain of the coracoclavicular ligaments. Palpation commonly reveals AC joint step-deformity.

III: Complete rupture of the AC ligament complex and the coracoclavicular ligaments, the coranoid and trapezoid. Palpation may reveal an increased AC step-deformity.

IV: Complete rupture of all ligaments with a posterior clavicular displacement resulting in increased signs of inflammation.

V: Complete rupture of all ligaments with significant superior displacement and a step-deformity of the elevated lateral clavicle compared to the acromion process. The coracoclavicular space can increase by 500% compared to the 25–100% of a type III injury.

VI: Complete rupture of all ligaments and an inferior clavicular displacement into the subacromial or subcoracoid cavity.

Treatment: Conservative treatment is recommended for type I and type II ACJ separations/sprains, type IV, V, VI are generally treated surgically and there is still some controversy surrounding the most appropriately method of treatment for a grade III [54, 108]. Some research does suggest that grade III should be treated conservatively first, and if unsuccessful then operative treatment can be considered, especially in the athletic population [108].

Conservative treatment includes an initial adherence to the POLICE protocol for the acute period and then immobilisation for a period (~1–3weeks) [108], ideally in an elevated position. Once pain has subsided and mobilisation can be tolerated active range of movement should be introduced [108, 109]. Progressive strength exercises should then be implemented started with isometric work including the scapular stabilisers; closed kinetic chain exercises should be focused on early and then followed by open kinetic chain and long-lever exercises [54, 110]. All rehabilitation should focus on good shoulder health and kinetic chain alignment. This can then be progressed to return to play activity in athlete focusing on plyometric activity and contact training no earlier than week 6 [108].

Scapular Dyskinesia

Mechanism of Injury: Scapular dyskinesia (SD) is described as abnormal scapular function during shoulder movement [111–112]. There are a multitude of factors that can result or contribute to SD: it has been known to be present in many shoulder diseases such as rotator cuff injury, GH joint instability, labral pathology and shoulder impingement and other chronic degenerative pathologies [112–115]. SD is also known to be a non-specific response to painful shoulder conditions; however, according to [116] this is opposed to specific GH joint pathology. One of the most common causes of SD is soft tissue alteration [114, 117]. When muscle imbalance occurs, and muscles that work to stabilise the glenohumeral and scapulothoracic joints become weakened or short in length, the position of the scapular changes, both during motion and at rest [112, 116]. Proper function of the glenohumeral joint requires a balanced activity of the scapular-stabilising muscles to allow the scapula to move on the posterolateral surface of the thoracic cage [118]. High risk groups include overhead athletes and those that use a computer for long periods of time [111].

Symptoms: SD can be observed during clinical evaluation of scapular motions during both shoulder movement and when static. According to Kibler [119] there are three classifications of SD:

Type 1/Inferior dysfunction: visual features are the prominence of the inferior angle of the scapular, resulting in an anterior tilt in the sagittal plane.

This pattern is most found in patients with rotator cuff dysfunction.

Type 2/Medial dysfunction: visual features are the prominence of the entire medial border of the scapular; this is due to internal rotation of the scapular in the transverse plane. Often occurs due to fatigue of the trapezius and rhomboids. Type 2 pattern mostly occurs in patients with GH joint instability.

Type 3/Superior dysfunction: visual features are excessive and early elevation of the scapular during elevation. Treatment: the main goal of treatment should be to rectify any imbalance of muscle, strengthening the weakened muscles and lengthening the shortened [111]; this may differ depending on the classification of SD. Focus should start with scapular control in a conscious state, with daily activity and then progress to during functional activity and sport performance [111]. Exercise should be completed with the focus of scapular pro-traction and depression and external shoulder rotation.

Elbow

Lateral Epicondylitis

Mechanism of Injury: Otherwise known as tennis elbow, lateral epicondylitis is a common, degen-erative tendinopathy [120]. It normally occurs due to activities that place stress on the wrist extensor muscles, for example the backhand in tennis, hence the name 'tennis elbow' [11]. These muscles attach at the lateral epicondyle region of the humerus; primarily the extensor carpi radialis brevis is involved [11, 120]. Lateral epicondylitis is common in upper extremity sports and activ-ities where combined elbow and wrist movements are elicited, such as swimming, racket sports, throwing events and wheelchair athletics [11, 120]. Along with this people that complete repeti-tive one-sided daily jobs such as the use of computers and manual labour often present with this condition. Due to these factors the dominant hand is usually most affected. There have also been some studies that have presented a relationship between lateral epicondylitis and dysfunction at the cervical, the shoulder and at the wrist joint/region [54].

Symptoms: The most common and prominent symptom is pain that comes on gradually over a period of time, located and often reproduced by palpation of the lateral epicondyle and the muscles at this attachment [11, 121–122]. Pain and weakness are present in wrist and finger extension and resisted supination [120]; however, some reports suggest the pain tends to be eased if the elbow is held in flexion [120]. Range of motion at the elbow is not normally affected; however, some pain can be elicited with the elbow in full extension with pronation of the forearm [44]. Wrist range of motion can sometimes present as deficient. It is not common to see inflammation at the lateral epicondyle; there is generally a very minimal inflammatory response [54]. As this is a tendon path-ology symptom may also present in line with the three-stage tendinopathy continuum presented by Cook and Purdam [6].

Treatment: Treatment for lateral epicondylitis is still not conclusive and is still widely researched and discussed. In the acute stage it is important to treat the symptoms and reduce the risk of further aggravation [54]. There are many proposed treatment methods listed below:

Physical therapy
Acupuncture
Soft tissue therapies
Non-steroidal anti-inflammatory drugs
Corticosteroid injections
Autologous blood injections
Platelet-rich plasma injections
Low-level laser therapy
Taping Techniques
Glyceryl Trinitrate patches
Shockwave therapy [120, 54].

Rehabilitation has shown positive outcomes for most patients[63]. Exercise-based rehabilitation should follow similar protocols to tendon rehab; there is no standardised rehab programme for lateral epicondylitis, but the principal should be to load the tendon appropriately and in a progressive manor [54]. Regaining strength in wrist flexion and extension, radial and ulnar deviation and grip strength are important. Strength can be first completed with isometrics before progression to eccentrics which are a favourable type of loading for tendon pathology.

It should be emphasised that a conservative approach with physical therapy, patient education and avoidance of aggravating activities should be the key message to both practitioners and patients.

Olecranon Bursitis

Mechanism of Injury: Olecranon bursitis is a common condition that is caused by acute or repetitive trauma to the bursa overlying the olecranon process at the proximal aspect of the ulna [123–124]. Acute bursitis occurs from either direct or prolonged trauma or pressure on the bursa [125]; when multiple episodes occur this can cause chronic bursitis. Other reasons for this type of bursitis are occupational or recreational activities that involve prolonged pressure on the bursa such as leaning on hard floors or rubbing on the elbow [125]. Other forms of bursitis include septic, which can be due to conditions such a gout or pseudogout [123–124, 126].

Symptoms: Patients often find swelling at the posterior elbow, sometimes recognisable as a goose egg over the olecranon process [123–124]. In some patients tenderness is present on palpation of the affected site; if infection is present, there may be warmth or redness present also. Range of motion is mostly unaffected; however, some patients suffer from pain during flexion and extension, particularly at end range of motion. This has been known to limit end range flexion in some patients [127].

Treatment: For most non-infection cases of bursitis, the condition is inflammatory, therefore conservative treatment methods focused on reducing inflammation have positive outcomes. If activity is an aggravating factor, then modification should be considered along with the use of padded splinting and patient education [126]. If patients do not respond or symptoms become chronic, aspiration can be considered with and without bandaging [127–129]. Other treatment methods include corticosteroid injections, and the use of non-steroidal anti-inflammatory medication.

For patients unresponsive to conservative management, surgical interventions can be considered which include removal of the inflamed bursa. Patients that take this route should then partake in rehabilitation post-surgery including strengthening and mobility exercises [128–129].

Hand

Scaphoid Fracture

Mechanism of Injury: The main cause of a fractured scaphoid is a fall on an outstretched arm/hand, often with a radially deviated wrist. This results in excessive extension of the wrist and compression of the hand. The applied force onto the scaphoid bone can cause a fracture [130–132] (Figure 3.7).

Symptoms: Patients may experience dull ache around the radial part of the wrist, pain or tenderness on palpation of the anatomical snuffbox along with tenderness of the scaphoid tubercle, particularly with passive movements. Tests such as the scaphoid compression test have mixed predictive factors in identifying a scaphoid fracture [131]. Periodic bruising and swelling/effusion around the wrist can also be present. Aggravating factors include pinching and gripping movements.

Treatment: As it is not uncommon for scaphoid fractures to go undetected, all suspected scaphoid fractures with positive clinical findings that have a negative radiograph should be followed up with further imaging after 7–14 days, especially if symptoms persist.

Acute management of a scaphoid fracture is immobilisation of both the wrist and thumb and assessment of union should be considered depending on location of fracture (distal third, middle third, proximal third) [133].

Rehabilitation: Rehabilitation will depend on the surgical method of treatment and/or cast. Early stages should focus on regaining range of movement at both the wrist and thumb, along with shoulder and elbow if restricted. Focus should then move on to strengthening the muscles in the upper extremity, utilisation of therapeutic putty and hand therapy balls are often helpful to resume full function.

Scaphoid Fracture

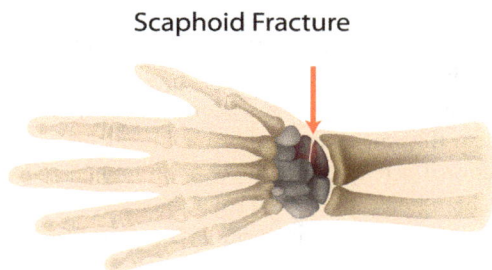

FIGURE 3.7 Scaphoid fracture.

Mallet Finger

Mechanism: Mallet finger is normally sustained from forced or excessive flexion of the distal interphalangeal (DIP) joint causing the extensor tendon to be stretched, torn or ruptured, and sometimes causing an avulsion of the tendon from the bone [134]. This injury often occurs from a forceful blow to the tip of the finger [135] and is common in athletes such as goalkeepers, basketball players and in sports that involve catching.

Symptoms: The main symptoms that present in mallet finger are pain in the effected joint and at the DIP joint. Deformity will often be present along with functional deficit resulting in the inability to actively extend the joint [136, 138].

Treatment: If left untreated mallet finger can cause long-term problems including osteoarthritis [136], and a 'swan neck' deformity. The majority of simple mallet finger injuries can be treated conservatively with rehabilitation and the use of a splint to immobilise the DIP joint alone. The splint should maintain full extension or slight hyperextension of the joint [3, 139, 134, 140], and should be splinted during the day for a minimum of six weeks followed by two weeks of night-time splinting [136]. It is important six weeks of splinting is completed; if it is interrupted, it should be restarted for optimal outcomes [137, 141]. Rehabilitation should focus on active flexion exercises to regain strength and functionality of the injured finger.

References

1. Brukner, P., & Khan, K. (2010). *Clinical sports medicine* (3rd ed). New Delhi: McGraw-Hill. https://blackwells.co.uk/bookshop/product/9780070278998
2. Challoumas, D., Kirwan, P. D., Borysov, D., Clifford, C., McLean, M., & Millar, N. L. (2019). Topical glyceryl trinitrate for the treatment of tendinopathies: a systematic review. *British journal of sports medicine, 53*(4), 251–262. https://doi.org/10.1136/bjsports-2018-099552
3. Comfort, P., & Abrahamson, E. (2010). *Sports rehabilitation and injury prevention.* Wiley-Blackwell https://www.wiley.com/en-gb/Sports+Rehabilitation+and+Injury+Prevention-p-9780470985632
4. Murphy, M. C., Travers, M. J., Chivers, P., Debenham, J. R., Docking, S. I., Rio, E. K., & Gibson, W. (2019). Efficacy of heavy eccentric calf training for treating mid-portion Achilles tendinopathy: a systematic review and meta-analysis. *British journal of sports medicine, 53*(17), 1070–1077. https://doi.org/10.1136/bjsports-2018-099934
5. Sprague, A. L., Smith, A. H., Knox, P., Pohlig, R. T., & Grävare Silbernagel, K. (2018). Modifiable risk factors for patellar tendinopathy in athletes: a systematic review and meta-analysis. *British journal of sports medicine, 52*(24), 1575–1585. https://doi.org/10.1136/bjsports-2017-099000
6. Cook, J. L., & Purdam, C. R. (2009). Is tendon pathology a continuum? A pathology model to explain the clinical presentation of load-induced tendinopathy. *British journal of sports medicine, 43*(6), 409–416. https://doi.org/10.1136/bjsm.2008.051193
7. Cook, J. L., Rio, E., Purdam, C. R., & Docking, S. I. (2016). Revisiting the continuum model of tendon pathology: what is its merit in clinical practice and research?. *British journal of sports medicine, 50*(19), 1187–1191. https://doi.org/10.1136/bjsports-2015-095422
8. Rio, E. K., McAuliffe, S., Kuipers, I., et al. (2020). ICON PART-T (2019)–International Scientific Tendinopathy Symposium Consensus: recommended standards for reporting participant characteristics in tendinopathy research (PART-T). *British journal of sports medicine 54*, 627–630 https://bjsm.bmj.com/content/54/11/627
9. van der Vlist, A. C., Winters, M., Weir, A., Ardern, C. L., Welton, N. J., Caldwell, D. M., Verhaar, J., & de Vos, R. J. (2020). Which treatment is most effective for patients with Achilles tendinopathy? A living systematic review with network meta-analysis of 29 randomised controlled trials. *British journal of sports medicine*, bjsports-2019–101872. Advance online publication. https://doi.org/10.1136/bjsports-2019–101872
10. Krey, D., Borchers, J., & McCamey, K. (2015). Tendon needling for treatment of tendinopathy: a systematic review. *The physician and sportsmedicine, 43*(1), 80–86. https://doi.org/10.1080/00913847.2015.1004296
11. Shultz, S., Houglum, P. A., & Perrin, D. H. (2010). *Examination of musculoskeletal injuries* (3rd ed). Champaign, IL: Human Kinetics. http://www.humankinetics.com/examinationofmusculoskeletal injuries
12. Dubois, B., Esculier, J. (2019). *Soft tissue injuries simply need PEACE & LOVE.* BJSM Blog, 2019. https://blogs.bmj.com/bjsm/2019/04/26/soft-tissue-injuries-simply-need-peace-love/
13. Gribble, P. A., Bleakley, C. M., Caulfield, B. M., et al. (2016). Evidence review for the 2016 International Ankle Consortium consensus statement on the prevalence, impact and long-term consequences of lateral ankle sprains. *British journal of sports medicine*, 50, 1496–1505. https://bjsm.bmj.com/content/50/24/1496
14. Hiller, C. E., Kilbreath, S. L., & Refshauge, K. M. (2011). Chronic ankle instability: evolution of the model. *Journal of athletic training, 46*(2), 133–141. https://doi.org/10.4085/1062-6050-46.2.133

15. Landrum, E. L., Kelln, B. M., Parente, W. R., Ingersoll, C. D., & Hertel, J. (2013). Immediate effects of anterior-to-posterior talocrural joint mobilization after prolonged ankle immobilization: a preliminary study. *Journal of manual & manipulative therapy, 16*(2), 100–105. 10.1179/106698108790818413

16. Hudson, R., Baker, R. T., May, J., Reordan, D., & Nasypany, A. (2017). Novel treatment of lateral ankle sprains using the Mulligan concept: an exploratory case series analysis. *The Journal of manual & manipulative therapy, 25*(5), 251–259. https://doi.org/10.1080/10669817.2017.1332557

17. Miklovic, T. M., Donovan, L., Protzuk, O. A., Kang, M. S., & Feger, M. A. (2018). Acute lateral ankle sprain to chronic ankle instability: a pathway of dysfunction. *The Physician and sportsmedicine, 46*(1), 116–122. https://doi.org/10.1080/00913847.2018.1409604

18. Petersen, W., Rembitzki, I. V., Koppenburg, A. G., Ellermann, A., Liebau, C., Brüggemann, G. P., & Best, R. (2013). Treatment of acute ankle ligament injuries: a systematic review. *Archives of orthopaedic and trauma surgery, 133*(8), 1129–1141. https://doi.org/10.1007/s00402-013-1742-5

19. Turnipseed, W. D., Hurschler, C., & Vanderby, R., Jr. (1995). The effects of elevated compartment pressure on tibial arteriovenous flow and relationship of mechanical and biochemical characteristics of fascia to genesis of chronic anterior compartment syndrome. *Journal of vascular surgery, 21*(5), 810–817. https://doi.org/10.1016/s0741-5214(05)80012–6

20. Drexler, M., Rutenberg, T. F., Rozen, N., Warschawski, Y., Rath, E., Chechik, O., Rachevsky, G., & Morag, G. (2017). Single minimal incision fasciotomy for the treatment of chronic exertional compartment syndrome: outcomes and complications. *Archives of orthopaedic and trauma surgery, 137*(1), 73–79. https://doi.org/10.1007/s00402-016-2569-7

21. Bong, M. R., Polatsch, D. B., Jazrawi, L. M., & Rokito, A. S. (2005). Chronic exertional compartment syndrome: diagnosis and management. *Bulletin (Hospital for Joint Diseases), 62*(3–4), 77–84.

22. Frink, M., Klaus, A. K., Kuther, G., Probst, C., Gosling, T., Kobbe, P., Hildebrand, F., Richter, M., Giannoudis, P. V., Krettek, C., & Pape, H. C. (2007). Long-term results of compartment syndrome of the lower limb in polytraumatised patients. *Injury, 38*(5), 607–613. https://doi.org/10.1016/j.injury.2006.12.021

23. Bengtsson, H., Ekstrand, J., & Hägglund, M. (2013). Muscle injury rates in professional football increase with fixture congestion: an 11-year follow-up of the UEFA Champions League injury study. *British journal of sports medicine, 47*(12), 743–747. https://doi.org/10.1136/bjsports-2013–092383

24. Hägglund, M., Waldén, M., & Ekstrand, J. (2013). Risk factors for lower extremity muscle injury in professional soccer: the UEFA Injury Study. *The American journal of sports medicine, 41*(2), 327–335. https://doi.org/10.1177/0363546512470634

25. Green, B., Lin, M., Schache, A. G., McClelland, J. A., Semciw, A. I., Rotstein, A., Cook, J., & Pizzari, T. (2020). Calf muscle strain injuries in elite Australian Football players: A descriptive epidemiological evaluation. *Scandinavian journal of medicine & science in sports, 30*(1), 174–184. https://doi.org/10.1111/sms.13552.

26. Green, B., & Pizzari, T. (2017). Calf muscle strain injuries in sport: a systematic review of risk factors for injury. *British journal of sports medicine, 51*(16), 1189–1194. https://doi.org/10.1136/bjsports-2016-097177

27. Bryan Dixon, J. (2009). Gastrocnemius vs. soleus strain: how to differentiate and deal with calf muscle injuries. *Current reviews in musculoskeletal medicine, 2*(2), 74–77. https://doi.org/10.1007/s12178-009-9045-8

28. Prakash, A., Entwisle, T., Schneider, M., Brukner, P., & Connell, D. (2018). Connective tissue injury in calf muscle tears and return to play: MRI correlation. *British journal of sports medicine, 52*(14), 929–933. https://doi.org/10.1136/bjsports-2017-098362

29. Bayer, M. L., Magnusson, S. P., Kjaer, M., & Tendon Research Group Bispebjerg (2017). Early versus delayed rehabilitation after acute muscle injury. *The New England journal of medicine, 377*(13), 1300–1301. https://doi.org/10.1056/NEJMc1708134

30. Mallo, J., & Dellal, A. (2012). Injury risk in professional football players with special reference to the playing position and training periodization. *The Journal of sports medicine and physical fitness, 52*(6), 631–638.

31. Riel, H., Cotchett, M., Delahunt, E., Rathleff, M. S., Vicenzino, B., Weir, A., & Landorf, K. B. (2017). Is 'plantar heel pain' a more appropriate term than 'plantar fasciitis'? Time to move on. *British journal of sports medicine, 51*(22), 1576–1577. https://doi.org/10.1136/bjsports-2017-097519

32. Thompson, J. V., Saini, S. S., Reb, C. W., & Daniel, J. N. (2014). Diagnosis and management of plantar fasciitis. *The Journal of the American Osteopathic Association, 114*(12), 900–906. https://doi.org/10.7556/jaoa.2014.177

33. Hicks, J. H. (1954). The mechanics of the foot. II. The plantar aponeurosis and the arch. *Journal of anatomy, 88*(1), 25–30.

34. Schepsis, A. A., Leach, R. E., & Gorzyca, J. (1991). Plantar fasciitis. Etiology, treatment, surgical results, and review of the literature. *Clinical orthopaedics and related research*, 266, 185–196.

35. Neufeld, S. K., & Cerrato, R. (2008). Plantar fasciitis: evaluation and treatment. *The Journal of the American Academy of Orthopaedic Surgeons, 16*(6), 338–346. https://doi.org/10.5435/00124635-200806000-00006

36. Whittaker, G. A., Munteanu, S. E., Menz, H. B., Tan, J. M., Rabusin, C. L., & Landorf, K. B. (2018). Foot orthoses for plantar heel pain: a systematic review and meta-analysis. *British journal of sports medicine, 52*(5), 322–328. https://doi.org/10.1136/bjsports-2016-097355

37. van Leeuwen, K. D., Rogers, J., Winzenberg, T., & van Middelkoop, M. (2016). Higher body mass index is associated with plantar fasciopathy/'plantar fasciitis': systematic review and meta-analysis of various clinical and imaging risk factors. *British journal of sports medicine, 50*(16), 972–981. https://doi.org/10.1136/bjsports-2015-094695

38. Sullivan, J., Pappas, E., & Burns, J. (2020). Role of mechanical factors in the clinical presentation of plantar heel pain: implications for management. *Foot, 42*, 101636. https://doi.org/10.1016/j.foot.2019.08.007

39. Rathleff, M. S., & Thorborg, K. (2015). 'Load me up, Scotty': mechanotherapy for plantar fasciopathy (formerly known as plantar fasciitis). *British journal of sports medicine, 49*(10), 638–639. https://doi.org/10.1136/bjsports-2014-094562

40. Petraglia, F., Ramazzina, I., & Costantino, C. (2017). Plantar fasciitis in athletes: diagnostic and treatment strategies. A systematic review. *Muscles, ligaments and tendons journal*, 7(1), 107–118. https://doi.org/10.11138/mltj/2017.7.1.107

41. Monteagudo, M., de Albornoz, P. M., Gutierrez, B., Tabuenca, J., & Álvarez, I. (2018). Plantar fasciopathy: a current concepts review. *EFORT open reviews, 3*(8), 485–493. https://doi.org/10.1302/2058-5241.3.170080

42. Thomas, J. L., Christensen, J. C., Kravitz, S. R., Mendicino, R. W., Schuberth, J. M., Vanore, J. V., Weil, L. S., Sr., Zlotoff, H. J., Bouché, R., Baker, J., & American College of Foot and Ankle Surgeons heel pain committee (2010). The diagnosis and treatment of heel pain: a clinical practice guideline-revision 2010. *The Journal of foot and ankle surgery: official publication of the American College of Foot and Ankle Surgeons, 49*(3 Suppl), S1–S19. https://doi.org/10.1053/j.jfas.2010.01.001

43. Hewett, T. E., Myer, G. D., & Ford, K. R. (2006). Anterior cruciate ligament injuries in female athletes: part 1, mechanisms and risk factors. *The American journal of sports medicine, 34*(2), 299–311. https://doi.org/10.1177/0363546505284183

44. Haim, A., Pritsch, T., Yosepov, L., & Arbel, R. (2006). *Harefuah, 145*(3), 208–245.

45. Lin, C. F., Gross, M., Ji, C., Padua, D., Weinhold, P., Garrett, W. E., & Yu, B. (2009). A stochastic biomechanical model for risk and risk factors of non-contact anterior cruciate ligament injuries. *Journal of biomechanics, 42*(4), 418–423. https://doi.org/10.1016/j.jbiomech.2008.12.005

46. Waldén, M., Krosshaug, T., Bjørneboe, J., Andersen, T. E., Faul, O., & Hägglund, M. (2015). Three distinct mechanisms predominate in non-contact anterior cruciate ligament injuries in male professional football players: a systematic video analysis of 39 cases. *British journal of sports medicine, 49*(22), 1452–1460. https://doi.org/10.1136/bjsports-2014-094573

47. Wetters, N., Weber, A., Wuerz, T., Schub, D., & Mandelbaum, B. (2015). Mechanism of injury and risk factors for anterior cruciate ligament injury. *Operative techniques in sports medicine*, 24. 10.1053/j.otsm.2015.09.001.

48. Hickey Lucas, K., Kline, P., Ireland, M., & Noehren, B. (2017). Hip and trunk muscle dysfunction: implications for anterior cruciate ligament injury prevention. *Annals of joint*, 2(5). http://aoj.amegroups.com/article/view/3676

49. Renstrom, P., Ljungqvist, A., Arendt, E., Beynnon, B., Fukubayashi, T., Garrett, W., Georgoulis, T., Hewett, T. E., Johnson, R., Krosshaug, T., Mandelbaum, B., Micheli, L., Myklebust, G., Roos, E., Roos, H., Schamasch, P., Shultz, S., Werner, S., Wojtys, E., & Engebretsen, L. (2008). Non-contact ACL injuries in

female athletes: an International Olympic Committee current concepts statement. *British journal of sports medicine, 42*(6), 394–412. https://doi.org/10.1136/bjsm.2008.048934

50. Herrington, L., & Fowler, E. (2006). A systematic literature review to investigate if we identify those patients who can cope with anterior cruciate ligament deficiency. *The Knee, 13*(4), 260–265. https://doi.org/10.1016/j.knee.2006.02.010

51. Kyritsis, P., Bahr, R., Landreau, P., Miladi, R., & Witvrouw, E. (2016). Likelihood of ACL graft rupture: not meeting six clinical discharge criteria before return to sport is associated with a four times greater risk of rupture. *British journal of sports medicine, 50*(15), 946–951. https://doi.org/10.1136/bjsports-2015-095908

52. Herrington, L., Myer, G., & Horsley, I. (2013). Task based rehabilitation protocol for elite athletes following Anterior Cruciate ligament reconstruction: a clinical commentary. *Physical therapy in sport: official journal of the Association of Chartered Physiotherapists in Sports Medicine, 14*(4), 188–198. https://doi.org/10.1016/j.ptsp.2013.08.001

53. Gokeler, A., Seil, R., Kerkhoffs, G., & Verhagen, E. (2018). A novel approach to enhance ACL injury prevention programs. *Journal of experimental orthopaedics, 5*(1), 22. https://doi.org/10.1186/s40634-018-0137-5

54. Ward, K. (Ed.). (2016). *Routledge handbook of sports therapy, injury assessment and rehabilitation*. London: Routledge. https://doi.org/10.4324/9780203807194

55. McAllister, D. R., & Petrigliano, F. A. (2007). Diagnosis and treatment of posterior cruciate ligament injuries. *Current sports medicine reports, 6*(5), 293–299.

56. Rigby, J., & Porter, K. (2010). Posterior cruciate ligament injuries. *Trauma*, 12(3), 175–181. https://doi.org/10.1177/1460408610378792

57. Margheritini, F., & Mariani, P. P. (2003). Diagnostic evaluation of posterior cruciate ligament injuries. *Knee surgery, sports traumatology, arthroscopy: official journal of the ESSKA, 11*(5), 282–288. https://doi.org/10.1007/s00167-003-0409-0

58. Agolley, D., Gabr, A., Benjamin-Laing, H., & Haddad, F. S. (2017). Successful return to sports in athletes following non-operative management of acute isolated posterior cruciate ligament injuries: medium-term follow-up. *The Bone & joint journal, 99-B*(6), 774–778. https://doi.org/10.1302/0301-620X.99B6.37953

59. Wang, D., Graziano, J., Williams, R. J. III, & Jones, K. J. (2018). Nonoperative treatment of PCL injuries: goals of rehabilitation and the natural history of conservative care. *Current reviews in musculoskeletal medicine, 11*(2), 290–297. https://doi.org/10.1007/s12178-018-9487-y

60. Andrews, K., Lu, A., Mckean, L., & Ebraheim, N. (2017). Review: medial collateral ligament injuries. *Journal of orthopaedics, 14*(4), 550–554. https://doi.org/10.1016/j.jor.2017.07.017

61. Melton, T. K. J., & Memarzadeh, A. (2019). Medial collateral ligament of the knee, anatomy, management, and surgical techniques for reconstruction. *Orthopaedics and trauma*, 33. https://doi.org/10.1016/j.mporth.2019.01.004

62. Elliott, M., & Johnson, D. L. (2015). Management of medial-sided knee injuries. *Orthopedics, 38*(3), 180–184. https://doi.org/10.3928/01477447-20150305-06

63. Hoogvliet, P., Randsdorp, M. S., Dingemanse, R., Koes, B. W., & Huisstede, B. M. (2013). Does effectiveness of exercise therapy and mobilisation techniques offer guidance for the treatment of lateral and medial epicondylitis? A systematic review. *British journal of sports medicine, 47*(17), 1112–1119. https://doi.org/10.1136/bjsports-2012-091990

64. Holden, S., & Rathleff, M. S. (2020). Separating the myths from facts: time to take another look at Osgood-Schlatter 'disease'. *British journal of sports medicine, 54*(14), 824–825. https://doi.org/10.1136/bjsports-2019-101888

65. Baltaci, G., Ozer, H., & Tunay, V. B. (2004). Rehabilitation of avulsion fracture of the tibial tuberosity following Osgood-Schlatter disease. *Knee surgery, sports traumatology, arthroscopy: official journal of the ESSKA, 12*(2), 115–118. https://doi.org/10.1007/s00167-003-0383-6

66. Kujala, U. M., Kvist, M., & Osterman, K. (1986). Knee injuries in athletes. Review of exertion injuries and retrospective study of outpatient sports clinic material. *Sports medicine, 3*(6), 447–460. https://doi.org/10.2165/00007256-198603060-00006

67. Çakmak, S., Tekin, L., & Akarsu, S. (2014). Long-term outcome of Osgood-Schlatter disease: not always favorable. *Rheumatology international, 34*(1), 135–136. https://doi.org/10.1007/s00296-012-2592-0

68. Bhatia Munisha, M. (2020). Osgood-Schlatter disease. *Emedicine* (e-journal). https://emedicine.medscape.com/article/1993268-overview

69. Wall, E. J. (1998). Osgood-schlatter disease: practical treatment for a self-limiting condition. *The Physician and sportsmedicine, 26*(3), 29–34. https://doi.org/10.3810/psm.1998.03.802

70. Soprano, J. V., & Fuchs, S. M. (2007). Common overuse injuries in the pediatric and adolescent athlete. *Clinical Pediatric Emergency Medicine, 8*(1), 7–14. https://doi.org/10.1016/j.cpem.2007.02.009

71. Kaya, D. O., Toprak, U., Baltaci, G., Yosmaoglu, B., & Ozer, H. (2013). Long-term functional and sono-graphic outcomes in Osgood-Schlatter disease. *Knee surgery, sports traumatology, arthroscopy: official journal of the ESSKA, 21*(5), 1131–1139. https://doi.org/10.1007/s00167-012-2116-1

72. Rathleff, M. S., Winiarski, L., Krommes, K., Graven-Nielsen, T., Hölmich, P., Olesen, J. L., Holden, S., & Thorborg, K. (2020). Pain, sports participation, and physical function in adolescents with patellofemoral pain and Osgood-Schlatter disease: a matched cross-sectional study. *The Journal of orthopaedic and sports physical therapy, 50*(3), 149–157. https://doi.org/10.2519/jospt.2020.8770

73. Ekstrand, J., Healy, J. C., Waldén, M., Lee, J. C., English, B., & Hägglund, M. (2012). Hamstring muscle injuries in professional football: the correlation of MRI findings with return to play. *British journal of sports medicine, 46*(2), 112–117. https://doi.org/10.1136/bjsports-2011-090155

74. Wing, C., & Bishop, C. (2020). Hamstring strain injuries: incidence, mechanisms, risk factors, and training recommendations. *Strength and conditioning journal, 42*(3), 40–57. 10.1519/SSC.0000000000000538

75. Liu, H., Garret, W. E., Moorman, C. T., & Yu, B. (2012). Injury rate, mechanism and risk factors of ham-string strain injury in sports: a review of literature. *Journal of sport and health science, 1*. https://doi.org/10.1016/j.jshs.

76. Timmins, R. G., Bourne, M. N., Shield, A. J., Williams, M. D., Lorenzen, C., & Opar, D. A. (2016). Short biceps femoris fascicles and eccentric knee flexor weakness increase the risk of hamstring injury in elite football (soccer): a prospective cohort study. *British journal of sports medicine, 50*(24), 1524–1535. https://doi.org/10.1136/bjsports-2015-095362. 0.

77. Vermeulen, R. (2019). What is a hamstring injury? An overview of anatomy, muscle healing and optimal loading. *Aspetar sports medicine journal.* https://www.aspetar.com/journal/upload/PDF/2019327121859.pdf

78. Van Dyk, N., & Whitely, R. (2015). Hamstring rehabilitation: criteria based progression protocol and clinical predictors for return to play. *BJSM Blog* https://blogs.bmj.com/bjsm/2015/11/22/hamstring-rehabilitation-criteria-based-progression-protocol-and-clinical-predictors-for-return-to-play

79. Valle, X., Tol, L. J., Hamilton, B., Rodas, G., Malliaras, P., Malliaropoulos, N., Rizo, V., Moreno, M., & Jardi, J. (2015). Hamstring muscle injuries, a rehabilitation protocol purpose. *Asian journal of sports medicine, 6*(4), e25411. https://doi.org/10.5812/asjsm.25411

80. Hartvigsen, J., Hancock, M. J., Kongsted, A., Louw, Q., Ferreira, M. L., Genevay, S., Hoy, D., Karppinen, J., Pransky, G., Sieper, J., Smeets, R. J., Underwood, M., & Lancet Low Back Pain Series Working Group (2018). What low back pain is and why we need to pay attention. *Lancet, 391*(10137), 2356–2367. https://doi.org/10.1016/S0140-6736(18)30480-X

81. Maher, C., Underwood, M., & Buchbinder, R. (2017). Non-specific low back pain. *Lancet, 389*(10070), 736–747. https://doi.org/10.1016/S0140-6736(16)30970–9

82. Nadler, S. F., Malanga, G. A., Bartoli, L. A., Feinberg, J. H., Prybicien, M., & Deprince, M. (2002). Hip muscle imbalance and low back pain in athletes: influence of core strengthening. *Medicine and science in sports and exercise, 34*(1), 9–16. https://doi.org/10.1097/00005768-200201000-00003

83. Burton, A. K., Tillotson, K. M., Main, C. J., & Hollis, S. (1995). Psychosocial predictors of out-come in acute and subchronic low back trouble. *Spine, 20*(6), 722–728. https://doi.org/10.1097/00007632-199503150-00014

84. Gillis, T S. (2019). Spondylolisthesis in sports. *International sportmed journal, StatPearls.*

85. Gallagher, B., Moatz, B., & Tortolani, P. J. (2020). Classifications in spondylolisthesis. *Seminars in spine sur-gery* [100802]. https://doi.org/10.1016/j.semss.2020.100802

86. Wicker, A. (2008). Spondylolysis and spondylolisthesis in sports. *International sportmed journal, 9*(2), 74–78. https://journals.co.za/content/ismj/9/2/EJC48630?fromSearch=true#abstract_content

87. Kalichman, L., Kim, D. H., Li, L., Guermazi, A., Berkin, V., & Hunter, D. J. (2009). Spondylolysis and spondylolisthesis: prevalence and association with low back pain in the adult community-based popula-tion. *Spine, 34*(2), 199–205. https://doi.org/10.1097/BRS.0b013e31818edcfd

88. Nava-Bringas, T. I., Ramírez-Mora, I., Coronado-Zarco, R., Macías-Hernández, S. I., Cruz-Medina, E., Arellano-Hernández, A., Hern Ndez-López, M., & León-Hernández, S. R. (2014). Association of strength, muscle balance, and atrophy with pain and function in patients with degenerative spondylolisthesis. *Journal of back and musculoskeletal rehabilitation, 27*(3), 371–376. https://doi.org/10.3233/BMR-140457.

89. Monticone, M., Ferrante, S., Teli, M., Rocca, B., Foti, C., Lovi, A., & Brayda Bruno, M. (2014). Management of catastrophising and kinesiophobia improves rehabilitation after fusion for lumbar spondylolisthesis and stenosis. A randomised controlled trial. *European spine journal: official publication of the European Spine Society, the European Spinal Deformity Society, and the European Section of the Cervical Spine Research Society, 23*(1), 87–95. https://doi.org/10.1007/s00586-013-2889-z

90. Wynne-Davies, R., & Scott, J. H. (1979). Inheritance and spondylolisthesis: a radiographic family survey. *The Journal of bone and joint surgery. British volume, 61-B*(3), 301–305. https://doi.org/10.1302/0301-620X.61B3.383720

91. Haun, D. W., & Kettner, N. W. (2005). Spondylolysis and spondylolisthesis: a narrative review of etiology, diagnosis, and conservative management. *Journal of chiropractic medicine, 4*(4), 206–217. https://doi.org/10.1016/S0899-3467(07)60153-0

92. MacAuley, D., & Best, T. (2007). *Evidence-based sports medicine* (2nd ed.). Blackwell Publishing. https://onlinelibrary.wiley.com/doi/book/10.1002/9780470988732

93. Standaert, C. J., & Herring, S. A. (2000). Spondylolysis: a critical review. *British journal of sports medicine, 34*(6), 415–422. https://doi.org/10.1136/bjsm.34.6.415

94. Grazina, R., Andrade, R., Santos, F. L., Marinhas, J., Pereira, R., Bastos, R., & Espregueira-Mendes, J. (2019). Return to play after conservative and surgical treatment in athletes with spondylolysis: A systematic review. *Physical therapy in sport: official journal of the Association of Chartered Physiotherapists in Sports Medicine, 37*, 34–43. https://doi.org/10.1016/j.ptsp.2019.02.005

95. Mataliotakis, G. I., & Tsirikos, A. I. (2017). Spondylolysis and spondylolisthesis in children and adolescents: current concepts and treatment. *Orthopaedics and trauma, 31*(6), 395–401. https://www.sciencedirect.com/science/article/abs/pii/S1877132717301070

96. Klouche, S., Lefevre, N., Herman, S., Gerometta, A., & Bohu, Y. (2016). Return to sport after rotator cuff tear repair: a systematic review and meta-analysis. *The American journal of sports medicine, 44*(7), 1877–1887. https://doi.org/10.1177/0363546515598995

97. Plate, J. F., Haubruck, P., Walters, J., Mannava, S., Smith, B. P., Smith, T. L., & Tuohy, C. J. (2013). Rotator cuff injuries in professional and recreational athletes. *Journal of surgical orthopaedic advances, 22*(2), 134–142. https://doi.org/10.3113/jsoa.2013.0134.

98. Lädermann, A., Denard, P. J., & Collin, P. (2015). Massive rotator cuff tears: definition and treatment. *International orthopaedics, 39*(12), 2403–2414. https://doi.org/10.1007/s00264-015-2796-5

99. Itoi, E. (2013). Rotator cuff tear: physical examination and conservative treatment. *Journal of orthopaedic science: official journal of the Japanese Orthopaedic Association, 18*(2), 197–204. https://doi.org/10.1007/s00776-012-0345-2.

100. Littlewood, C., Rangan, A., Beard, D. J., Wade, J., Cookson, T., & Foster, N. E. (2018). The enigma of rotator cuff tears and the case for uncertainty. *British journal of sports medicine, 52*(19), 1222. https://doi.org/10.1136/bjsports-2018-099063

101. Ranebo, M. C., Björnsson Hallgren, H. C., Holmgren, T., & Adolfsson, L. E. (2020). Surgery and physiotherapy were both successful in the treatment of small, acute, traumatic rotator cuff tears: a prospective randomized trial. *Journal of shoulder and elbow surgery, 29*(3), 459–470. https://doi.org/10.1016/j.jse.2019.10.013

102. Walch, G., Boileau, P., Noel, E., & Donell, S. T. (1992). Impingement of the deep surface of the supraspinatus tendon on the posterosuperior glenoid rim: an arthroscopic study. *Journal of shoulder and elbow surgery, 1*(5), 238–245. https://doi.org/10.1016/S1058-2746(09)80065-7

103. Ellenbecker, T. S., & Cools, A. (2010). Rehabilitation of shoulder impingement syndrome and rotator cuff injuries: an evidence-based review. *British journal of sports medicine, 44*(5), 319–327. https://doi.org/10.1136/bjsm.2009.058875

104. Diercks, R., Bron, C., Dorrestijn, O., Meskers, C., Naber, R., de Ruiter, T., Willems, J., Winters, J., van der Woude, H. J., & Dutch Orthopaedic Association (2014). Guideline for diagnosis and treatment of

subacromial pain syndrome: a multidisciplinary review by the Dutch Orthopaedic Association. *Acta orthopaedica, 85*(3), 314–322. https://doi.org/10.3109/17453674.2014.920991

105. Dong, W., Goost, H., Lin, X. B., Burger, C., Paul, C., Wang, Z. L., Zhang, T. Y., Jiang, Z. C., Welle, K., & Kabir, K. (2015). Treatments for shoulder impingement syndrome: a PRISMA systematic review and network meta-analysis. *Medicine, 94*(10), e510. https://doi.org/10.1097/MD.0000000000000510

106. Escamilla, R. F., Hooks, T. R., & Wilk, K. E. (2014). Optimal management of shoulder impingement syndrome. *Open access journal of sports medicine, 5*, 13–24. https://doi.org/10.2147/OAJSM.S36646

107. Heron, S. R., Woby, S. R., & Thompson, D. P. (2017). Comparison of three types of exercise in the treatment of rotator cuff tendinopathy/shoulder impingement syndrome: A randomized controlled trial. *Physiotherapy, 103*(2), 167–173. https://doi.org/10.1016/j.physio.2016.09.001

108. van Bergen, C., van Bemmel, A. F., Alta, T., & van Noort, A. (2017). New insights in the treatment of acromioclavicular separation. *World journal of orthopedics, 8*(12), 861–873. https://doi.org/10.5312/wjo.v8.i12.861

109. Graham, P. (2020). Acromioclavicular separation. *Orthopedic nursing, 39*(3), 201–203. https://doi.org/10.1097/NOR.0000000000000658

110. Reid, D., Polson, K., & Johnson, L. (2012). Acromioclavicular joint separations grades I–III: a review of the literature and development of best practice guidelines. *Sports medicine, 42*(8), 681–696. https://doi.org/10.2165/11633460-000000000-00000

111. Panagiotopoulos, A. C., & Crowther, I. M. (2019). Scapular dyskinesia, the forgotten culprit of shoulder pain and how to rehabilitate. *SICOT-J, 5*, 29. https://doi.org/10.1051/sicotj/2019029

112. Longo, U. G., Risi Ambrogioni, L., Berton, A., Candela, V., Massaroni, C., Carnevale, A., Stelitano, G., Schena, E., Nazarian, A., DeAngelis, J., & Denaro, V. (2020). Scapular dyskinesis: from basic science to ultimate treatment. *International journal of environmental research and public health, 17*(8), 2974. https://doi.org/10.3390/ijerph17082974

113. Huang, T. S., Ou, H. L., Huang, C. Y., & Lin, J. J. (2015). Specific kinematics and associated muscle activation in individuals with scapular dyskinesis. *Journal of shoulder and elbow surgery, 24*(8), 1227–1234. https://doi.org/10.1016/j.jse.2014.12.022

114. Kibler, W. B., Sciascia, A., & Wilkes, T. (2012). Scapular dyskinesis and its relation to shoulder injury. *The Journal of the American Academy of Orthopaedic Surgeons, 20*(6), 364–372. https://doi.org/10.5435/JAAOS-20-06-364

115. Carnevale, A., Longo, U. G., Schena, E., Massaroni, C., Lo Presti, D., Berton, A., Candela, V., & Denaro, V. (2019). Wearable systems for shoulder kinematics assessment: a systematic review. *BMC musculoskeletal disorders, 20*(1), 546. https://doi.org/10.1186/s12891-019-2930-4

116. Kibler, W. B., & Sciascia, A. (2010). Current concepts: scapular dyskinesis. *British journal of sports medicine, 44*(5), 300–305. https://doi.org/10.1136/bjsm.2009.058834

117. Kibler, W. B., & Sciascia, A. (2016). The role of the scapula in preventing and treating shoulder instability. *Knee surgery, sports traumatology, arthroscopy: official journal of the ESSKA, 24*(2), 390–397. https://doi.org/10.1007/s00167-015-3736-z

118. Merolla, G., De Santis, E., Campi, F., Paladini, P., & Porcellini, G. (2010). Supraspinatus and infraspinatus weakness in overhead athletes with scapular dyskinesis: strength assessment before and after restoration of scapular musculature balance. *Musculoskeletal surgery, 94*(3), 119–125. https://doi.org/10.1007/s12306-010-0082-7

119. Kibler, W. B., Uhl, T. L., Maddux, J. W., Brooks, P. V., Zeller, B., & McMullen, J. (2002). Qualitative clinical evaluation of scapular dysfunction: a reliability study. *Journal of shoulder and elbow surgery, 11*(6), 550–556. https://doi.org/10.1067/mse.2002.126766

120. Vaquero-Picado, A., Barco, R., & Antuña, S. A. (2017). Lateral epicondylitis of the elbow. *EFORT open reviews, 1*(11), 391–397. https://doi.org/10.1302/2058-5241.1.000049

121. Whaley, A. L., & Baker, C. L. (2004). Lateral epicondylitis. *Clinics in sports medicine, 23*(4), 677–x. https://doi.org/10.1016/j.csm.2004.06.004

122. Pienimäki, T., Tarvainen, T., Siira, P., Malmivaara, A., & Vanharanta, H. (2002). Associations between pain, grip strength, and manual tests in the treatment evaluation of chronic tennis elbow. *The Clinical journal of pain, 18*(3), 164–170. https://doi.org/10.1097/00002508-200205000-00005

123. Foye, P. M. (2010). Olecranon bursitis. *Medscape.*

124. Foye, P. M. (2009). Physical medicine and rehabilitation for olecranon bursitis. *Medscape*.

125. Larson, R. L., & Osternig, L. R. (1974). Traumatic bursitis and artificial turf. *The Journal of sports medicine, 2*(4), 183–188. https://doi.org/10.1177/036354657400200401

126. Herrera, F. A., & Meals, R. A. (2011). Chronic olecranon bursitis. *The Journal of hand surgery, 36*(4), 708–710. https://doi.org/10.1016/j.jhsa.2010.12.030

127. Reilly, D., & Kamineni, S. (2016). Olecranon bursitis. *Journal of shoulder and elbow surgery, 25*(1), 158–167. https://doi.org/10.1016/j.jse.2015.08.032.

128. Fisher, R. H. (1977). Conservative treatment of distended patellar and olecranon bursae. *Clinical orthopaedics and related research*, 123, 98. https://doi.org/10.1097/00003086-197703000-00035

129. Del Buono, A., Franceschi, F., Palumbo, A., Denaro, V., & Maffulli, N. (2012). Diagnosis and management of olecranon bursitis. *The surgeon: journal of the Royal Colleges of Surgeons of Edinburgh and Ireland, 10*(5), 297–300. https://doi.org/10.1016/j.surge.2012.02.002

130. Gutierrez, G. (1996). Office management of scaphoid fractures. *The Physician and sportsmedicine, 24*(8), 60–70. https://doi.org/10.3810/psm.1996.08.1379

131. Phillips, T. G., Reibach, A. M., & Slomiany, W. P. (2004). Diagnosis and management of scaphoid fractures. *American family physician, 70*(5), 879–884.

132. MacDermid, J. C., Turgeon, T., Richards, R. S., Beadle, M., & Roth, J. H. (1998). Patient rating of wrist pain and disability: a reliable and valid measurement tool. *Journal of orthopaedic trauma, 12*(8), 577–586. https://doi.org/10.1097/00005131-199811000-00009

133. Hayat, Z., & Varacallo, M. (2020). *Scaphoid wrist fracture*. StatPearls Publishing. https://www.ncbi.nlm.nih.gov/books/NBK536907.

134. Alla, S. R., Deal, N. D., & Dempsey, I. J. (2014). Current concepts: mallet finger. *Hand, 9*(2), 138–144. https://doi.org/10.1007/s11552-014-9609-y

135. Cheung, J. P., Fung, B., & Ip, W. Y. (2012). Review on mallet finger treatment. *Hand surgery: an international journal devoted to hand and upper limb surgery and related research: journal of the Asia-Pacific Federation of Societies for Surgery of the Hand, 17*(3), 439–447. https://doi.org/10.1142/S0218810412300033

136. Lamaris, G. A., & Matthew, M. K. (2017). The diagnosis and management of mallet finger injuries. *Hand, 12*(3), 223–228. https://doi.org/10.1177/1558944716642763

137. Bloom, J. M., Khouri, J. S., & Hammert, W. C. (2013). Current concepts in the evaluation and treatment of mallet finger injury. *Plastic and reconstructive surgery, 132*(4), 560e–566e. https://doi.org/10.1097/PRS.0b013e3182a0148c

138. Stack, H. G. (1969). Mallet finger. *Hand, 1*(2), 83–89. https://doi.org/10.1016/0072-968X(69)90069-2

139. Katzman, B. M., Klein, D. M., Mesa, J., Geller, J., & Caligiuri, D. A. (1999). Immobilization of the mallet finger. Effects on the extensor tendon. *Journal of hand surgery, 24*(1), 80–84. https://doi.org/10.1016/s0266-7681(99)90041-4

140. Tolkien, Z., Potter, S., Burr, N., Gardiner, M. D., Blazeby, J. M., Jain, A., & Henderson, J. (2017). Conservative management of mallet injuries: a national survey of current practice in the UK. *Journal of plastic, reconstructive & aesthetic surgery: JPRAS, 70*(7), 901–907. https://doi.org/10.1016/j.bjps.2017.04.009

141. Smit, J. M., Beets, M. R., Zeebregts, C. J., Rood, A., & Welters, C. F. (2010). Treatment options for mallet finger: a review. *Plastic and reconstructive surgery, 126*(5), 1624–1629. https://doi.org/10.1097/PRS.0b013e3181ef8ec8

4

PITCH-SIDE CARE

Ebony Fewkes and Mark Adamoulas

Taping

Sports taping is a method commonly used in sports to treat acute injuries as well as within the early stages of rehabilitation and return to play. Taping is used in order to restrict range of motion, protect a joint, improve stabilisation and proprioception and to reduce the risk of re- injury [1]. Over the years there have been many suggested techniques, all of which can be modified clinically to meet the athlete's individual needs.

When applying tape there are a few basic principles to adhere to:

- Use ridged tape to restrict range of motion
- Elastic tapes can be used to cover the ridged taping or for compression
- Apply anchors above and below the joint for the tape to attach to, ensuring these are not restrictive of the muscle movement
- Ensure the athlete is not allergic to any tapes or adhesive sprays, under-wrap may be applied if needed

Athletic Taping Techniques

Lateral Ankle

1. Position the client's foot in neutral
2. Using ridged tape, apply anchors around the mid-foot and the calf, superior to the malleoli
3. Starting on from the medial aspect of the calf anchor, apply a stirrup over the medial malleolus, under the heel, pulling up over the lateral malleolus attaching to the lateral aspect of the calf anchor
4. Apply a second stirrup, overlapping the tape by half
5. Apply a third stirrup if required
6. Apply a heel lock starting at the medial stirrup attachment, wind laterally around the anterior leg and continue posteriorly around the Achilles, under the calcaneus, back over the lateral ankle, over the anterior leg returning to the starting point
7. Secure the tape by re-applying both anchors (Figure 4.1)

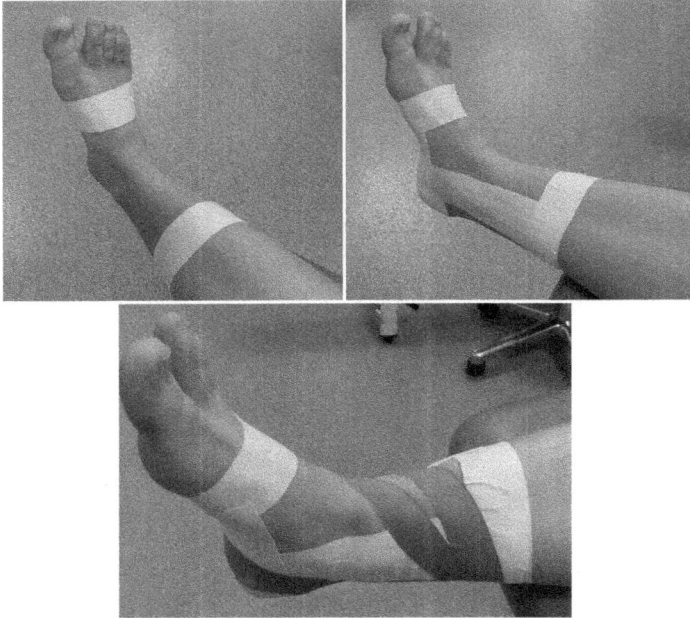

FIGURE 4.1 Lateral ankle taping method.

Alternate Heel Lock Technique

In addition to heel lock technique described above an alternative technique may be substituted.

Starting on the medial aspect of the mid-foot anchor, tape a 'U' around the heel at the lateral aspect of the mid-foot anchor.

Arch

1. Using ridged tape, apply tape from the lateral sole of the foot, under the foot medially, pulling up and over the dorsal aspect of the foot
2. Apply a second over lapping strip of tape
3. Re-enforce with further layering or a more ridged tape

Medial Knee

1. Position the knee in approximately 10 degrees of flexion
2. Using ridged tape, apply an anchor above and below the knee joint
3. Apply an X, distal to proximal, crossing the medial joint line
4. Re-enforce the X, overlapping the tape by half
5. Apply a third layer if required
6. Re-apply both anchors
7. Secure by applying elastic tape over the top (Figure 4.2) [2]

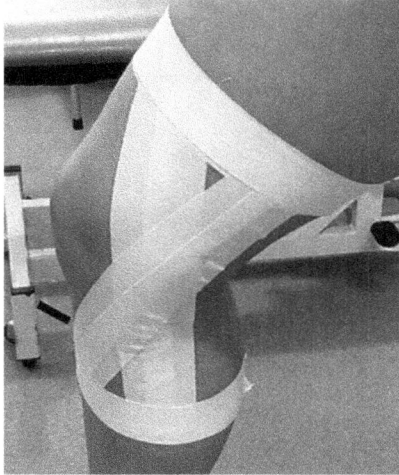

FIGURE 4.2   Medial knee taping method.

Lateral Knee

Following the same protocol as the medial knee support, applying the 'X' on the lateral side of the knee.

Cruciate Ligament or Meniscus Protection

Following the above knee taping principle, apply strapping to both the medial and lateral aspects of the knee to protect intra-articular structures. An 'X' may also be applied over the posterior knee to prevent hyperextension.

Patella Alignment

1. Using ridged tape apply an anchor over the patella, from medial to lateral, with no tension
2. For a medially deviated patella, using ridged tape apply over the anchor from medial to lateral, applying tension to secure the patella in the correct alignment
3. For a laterally deviated patella, using ridged tape apply over the anchor from lateral to medial, applying tension to secure the patella in the correct alignment [3]

Elbow Hyperextension

1. Position the elbow in 30-degree flexion
2. Using ridged tape, apply anchor above and below the elbow joint
3. Apply an X, distal to proximal, over the anterior elbow joint
4. Re-enforce the X, overlapping the tape by half
5. Apply a third layer if required
6. A small loop can be added around the centre of the cross if desired
7. Re-apply both anchors
8. Secure by applying elastic tape over top (Figure 4.3)

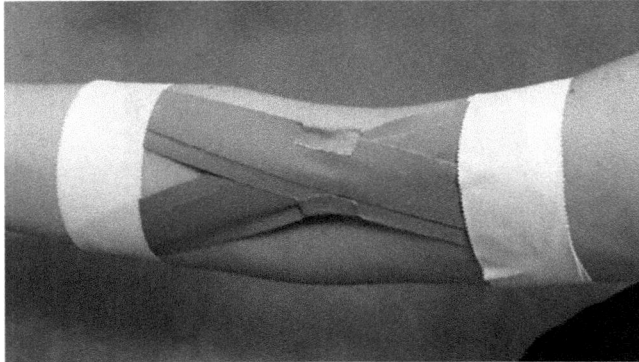

FIGURE 4.3 Elbow hyperextension taping method.

Shoulder Cuff or ACJ Taping

1. Position the athlete with their hand on their hip
2. Using ridged tape apply an anchor around the humerus
3. Apply a strip of tape anterior to posterior over the upper traps, proximal to the acromion clavicular joint (ACJ)
4. Apply and X from distal anchor to proximal anchor, forming a gap around the ACJ
5. A line of tape may be applied from the distal anchor directly up and over the ACJ for re-enforcement
6. Re-enforce, overlapping the tape by half, maintaining gap in tape over the ACJ
7. Apply a third layer if required
8. Re-apply both anchors
9. Secure by applying elastic tape over top (Figure 4.4)

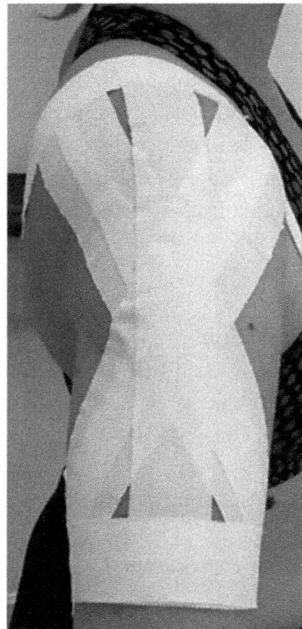

FIGURE 4.4 Shoulder cuff taping method.

Thumb Spica

1. Using ridged tape, apply an anchor around the wrist
2. Starting on the dorsal surface, apply the tape up over the dorsal thumb, wrap around the base of the thumb and back down to attach to the ventral aspect of the anchor
3. Re-enforce overlapping the tape by half as many times as required
4. Apply elastic tape from the dorsal aspect of wrist, around the base of the thumb, down to the ventral wrist
5. Continue back around the wrist and thumb as many times as required

Kinesio Taping Techniques

Kinesio tape was developed by Dr Kenzo Kase in the 1970s, since then, despite conflicting research evidence in regards to its effects, the anecdotal evidence for its use has been positive leading to it becoming used widely within both professional and amateur sporting environments. One of the benefits over traditional sports tape, is that Kinesio tape may remain on for 5–7days following application.

Kinesio tape is an elastic tape applied to a backing sheet with a normal tension of 10–20% stretch depending on the brand, which can stretch up to 120–140% of its length and is suggested to have many benefits including increasing blood flow, muscle activation, decreasing pain, decreasing swelling and inflammation, as well as supporting injured muscles and joints without unnecessarily restricting range of motion [4]. It is proposed that these effects arise from the tape 'lifting' the cutaneous layer of skin and fascia, decompressing the underlying tissue, as well as providing stimulus to the various mechanoreceptors within the cutaneous layer.

Muscle Activation and Inhibition

Kinesio tape can be applied to inhibit activity and relieve pain following a muscle strain or alternatively to activate an inhibited muscle during exercise. The target muscle should be placed on a pain free stretch before taping, tape ends should be rounded to prevent lifting and each end of the tape should be applied as an anchor with 0% or paper off stretch tension. When preparing the tape, rounding the edges will prevent any peeling and allow the application to remain for a longer period of time.

Muscle Activation: Apply the tape in the direction of origin to insertion with light tension (15%–25%) [5]).

Muscle Inhibition: Apply the tape in the direction of insertion to origin with light tension (15–25%) [6]). In addition, a pain strip, sometimes referred to as a 'zapper', may be applied transversely over the specific area of pain for effective pain relief with a high tension of 75%.

Achilles Tape

1. Place the foot in pain free dorsiflexion
2. Apply an anchor under the calcaneus
3. Attach the tape with light tension up the centre of the calf
4. Apply a high-tension zapper across the area of pain (Figure 4.5)

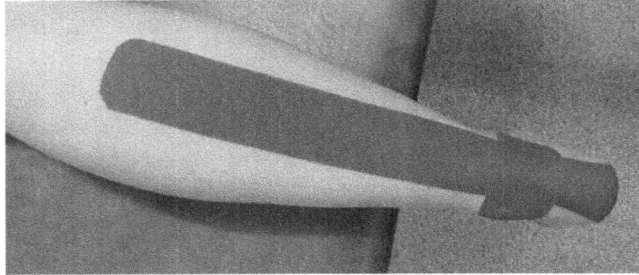

FIGURE 4.5   Achilles Kinesio taping method.

★Tape may be cut into a Y to allow coverage of both medial and lateral aspects of the calf★

Patella Offload

1. Seat the client with knees over the end of the plinth
2. Starting at the tibial tuberosity, apply a strip of light tension tape around the medial aspect of the patella, up into the quadriceps
3. Apply a second strip of light tension tape starting at the tibial tuberosity around the lateral aspect of the patella, up into the quadriceps
4. Apply a Zapper with high tension over the patella tendon for pain relief if required (Figure 4.6)

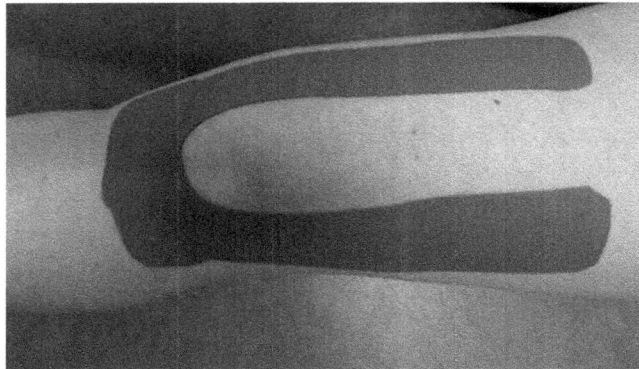

FIGURE 4.6   Patella offload Kinesio taping method.

Lower Back Pain

1. Place the athlete in a position of lumber flexion
2. Apply a strip of light tension tape from the SIJ up the back, parallel with the spine, on either side
3. Apply a Zapper with high tension over the area of pain for pain relief if required (Figure 4.7)

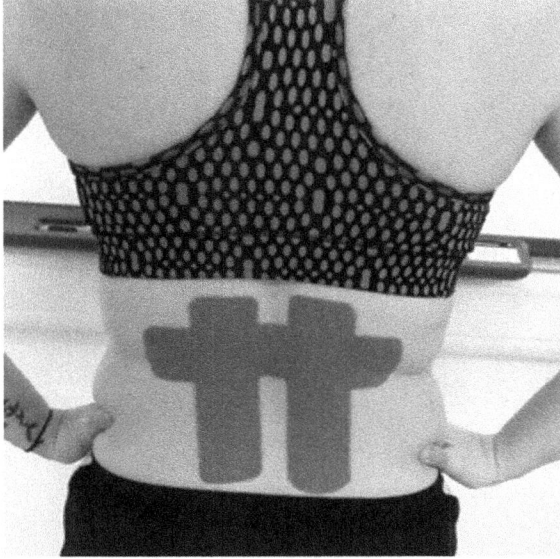

FIGURE 4.7   Lower back pain Kinesio taping method.

Posture

Kinesio tape can be used to address postural dysfunctions, by providing cutaneous stimulation and feedback, allowing the individual to maintain correct posture especially when muscles are fatigued [7]. In order for this to be effective the tape must 'pull' on the skin when the individual reverts to their incorrect posture, therefore it should be applied with high tension, approximately 75%.

Shoulder

1. Place the athlete in scapular retraction
2. Place an anchor anterior of the acromioclavicular joint
3. Apply tape with a high tension (75%) diagonally towards the inferior angle of the opposite scapular
4. Apply a strip of tape from the opposite side, creating an X between the scapular

Arch

1. Apply tape from the lateral sole of the foot, under the foot medially with medium tension, then pulling and over the dorsal aspect of the foot with high tension
2. Apply a second strip of tape next to the first

Lymphatic Drainage

Kinesio tape is commonly used to facilitate the healing of both haematomas and oedema. In this method the decompression effect of the tape is utilised in order to increase blood flow to the tissue [8] which in turn improves the efficiency of the lymphatic system in clearing waste from the injured area. The tape is applied with a light tension into 'fingers' which not only decompress

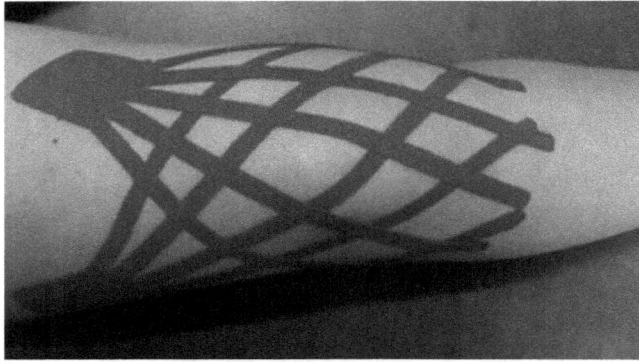

FIGURE 4.8 Lymphatic drainage Kinesio taping method.

the underlying tissue, but they also create a pressure gradient within the surrounding tissue allowing improved efficiency of lymphatic drainage.

1. Cut the tape to have an anchor and several 'fingers'
2. Apply and anchor of light or paper off tension at the edge of the injured area, pointing towards to closest lymph nodes
3. Apply the 'fingers' one at a time, with a light tension (25%) over the injury site, leaving space between each 'finger'. A second strip of tape may be applied in the above manner so that the 'fingers' create a mesh effect (Figure 4.8)

First Aid

As the medic responsible in a pitch-side environment it is essential that you are prepared with the knowledge and equipment to deal with any injury within a pre-hospital setting. Within this section we will outline the basic equipment which should be carried within your first aid kit, as well as the various first aid mnemonic's to assist you with your primary survey[9] and secondary survey[10].

As the medic responsible it is also essential that you know the location of the nearest appropriate emergency department and maintain updated emergency action plans and athlete records.

Equipment

When working as a first responder pitch side you need to ensure you carry the required equipment to help you deal with any situation that may arise. Essential equipment includes:

Gloves
Sterile dressing
Transpore tape
Sports tape
Clinical waste bag
Ice packs
Spinal board
Triangular bandage
Oropharyngeal airway (various sizes)

I-Gel supraglottic airway (various sizes)
Rescuer manual suction pump
Non-rebreathing mask (adult & paediatric)
Gauze
Wound cleansing wipes
Waterproof tape
Compression tape
Scissors
SAM splints
Laerdal stifneck select collar
Curaplex pocket mask
Nasopharyngeal airway (various sizes)
Lubricating jelly (42g tube)
Bag valve mask (adult)
Diagnostic penlight
Blood pressure cuff
Dual-head stethoscope

You should have easy access to a portable Automatic Emergency Defibrillator.

Initial Response

Shout for help
Assess the scene
Free from danger
Evaluate the player

Primary Survey

Your primary survey should follow the below systematic process in all casualties [9].

Safe Approach

- Is the scene safe for you to approach?
- Are you free from danger?

Airway

- Can they talk?
- Are there any obvious obstructions in the airway?

Breathing

- Look for chest raising
- Feel for breath on your cheek
- Listen for breathing sounds

Circulation

- Can you locate a radial pulse?
- What is the rate, rhythm, volume and character?
- Any visible catastrophic bleeding?

Disability

- Are they conscious?
- Think AVPU
  - Awake
  - Responds to verbal stimuli
  - Responds to pain stimuli
  - Unresponsive

Environment and Exposure

- Are there any other obvious injuries?
- How will they be extricated?
- If they are unable to be removed how can you prevent them from deteriorating?

Secondary Survey

Whilst waiting for emergency services to arrive it is essential you continue to monitor the athlete for any signs of deterioration. This can be done by monitoring their pulse rate and regularly repeating your ABCD. If suitably trained, you may be able to perform a more comprehensive secondary survey in including auscultation and percussion [10].

Handover to Emergency Services

For all athletes under your care it is advisable that you create SAMPLE cards to be held within their medical record, this allows essential information to be passed on to emergency services [11]. A SAMPLE card should include:

Signs and symptoms
Allergies
Medications
Past medical history
Last meal and drink
Event causing injury

Whilst several mnemonics exist for a patient handover, ATMIST is widely used and recognised within the health care industry [12]. The following information should be provided:

Age and gender
Time of incident and ETA
Mechanism of injury

Injury suspected
Signs and symptoms
Treatment

Immobilising

Appropriate identification and management of fracture and dislocation injuries is essential to reduce the risk of further health implications [13]. Following a systematic approach, any intervention to musculoskeletal injuries should occur as part of the primary survey [14]. With the exception of catastrophic bleeding, these injuries will be covered under 'E' environment and exposure. If available, all significant musculoskeletal injuries such as fractures and dislocations should be treated with high flow oxygen. Analgesia may also be issued by a suitably qualified professional.

Splints

There are various types of splints that may be used to immobilise injuries, some of the more commonly found splints include Sam splints, box splints and vacuum splints. The size of the splint used will depend on the suspected fracture location, ideally the joint above and below should be secured to prevent any unwanted movement.

Splint Application

1. It is essential that you first make an assessment of the injured limbs vascular status, this can be done by locating any pulse distal to the suspected injury location.
   ★Tip★ once a pulse has been located mark its location with a pen so that it can be located again with ease
2. Should the limb not be in the correct anatomical position you may be required to realign the limb before splinting, this can be done with the use of gentle traction
3. The vascular integrity of the limb should be checked following any realignment and following the application of the splint
4. Should you be unable to re-locate a distal pulse following realignment you should attempt to return the limb to its original position to re-establish the blood flow. In this situation the limb should be immobilised as much as possible until emergency services arrive
5. To apply the splint gently lift the limb, stabilising above and below the suspected fracture location, slide the splint underneath and gently lower the limb back down, secure the splint tightly
6. Vascular status should be monitored and any abnormalities should be highlighted to emergency services as this requires urgent care.

Triangle Bandage

In addition to splits, a triangle bandages may be used to immobilise the upper limb following trauma. There are two main techniques that may be used, the elevated sling and the more commonly used broad sling.

Broad Sling

The most commonly used sling for upper limb injuries is the broad sling, which can be used to immobilise shoulder, elbow and wrist injuries. Before splinting ensure you are able to locate a distal pulse.

1. Support the arm into a 90/90 position, parallel to the ground
2. Insert the bandage between the arm and the body, with the 'point' under the elbow and the upper end over the shoulder of the injured side
3. Bring the lower end up over the arm, over the opposite shoulder, and round the posterior of the neck
4. Tie together, ensuring the knot is located over the injured side shoulder
5. Tie the corner located at the elbow to ensure it is supported
6. Re-check for a distal pulse

Elevated Sling

This type of sling is commonly used to treat hand or finger injuries which require elevation to reduce swelling.

1. Support the arm so that the injured hand is on elevated on the opposite shoulder
2. Apply the bandage over the arm with the 'point' under the elbow and the upper end over the shoulder of the uninjured side
3. Fold the lower end of the bandage under the elbow, bringing the point around the back of the patient, ending at the posterior of the uninjured shoulder
4. Tie both ends together
5. Tie the corner located at the elbow to ensure it is supported

Suspected Spinal Injuries

In the case of the suspected spinal injury it is vital that you immobilise the athlete to prevent any further damage from occurring [15]. If necessary, they will need to be extracted from the pitch via spinal board. As first responder it will be you and your clinical assessment which determines how the player may be removed from the pitch. This decision will be based on the mechanism of injury, and your initial assessment [15]. If the athlete is alert and there is no indication of a spinal injury on assessment, it may be possible to clear the neck allowing the athlete to walk off the pitch. If the athlete is not alert or shows any signs of concussion and impaired understanding you will be unable to clear the neck, and therefore will need to be extracted via spinal board.

Spinal Board Extraction

1. Ensure it is safe to approach
2. Immobilise the athlete's neck with an anterior hold
3. Once the neck is secured speak to the athlete to determine if they are conscious
4. Shout for help and request an ambulance to be called
5. Ask an assistant to stabilise the neck with manual in line stabilisation (MILS)
6. Check your ABCD, maintaining MILS at all times

7. Measure the athlete's neck for collar size (upper trapezius to the chin)
8. Apply the collar, ensuring MILS is maintained throughout
9. Five people will be required to place the athlete on the scoop board, or 6 for a split board
10. Arrange the three helpers to log roll in height order – tallest at the head
11. Instruct them to place their hands in the required positions on the shoulder, hips, thigh and ankle (think 3 over, 3 under)
12. SPLIT BOARD
    a. On instruction of the person maintaining MILS roll the athlete to 15 degrees
    b. Insert one side of the board
    c. Again, on the count of the person maintaining MILS roll the athlete back down
    d. Walking around the feet of the athlete the log rollers need to position themselves in the same arrangement
    e. Roll the athlete to 15 degrees and insert the other side of the board, attaching them together before rolling the athlete back down
13. SCOOP BOARD
    a. On instruction of the person maintaining MILS roll the athlete to 90 degrees
    b. Insert the board
    c. Again, on the count of the person maintaining MILS roll the athlete back down
    d. Helpers will need to adjust their hand positioning to the shoulders, knees and ankles
    e. On the instruction of the person in MILS reposition the athlete onto the board
14. If the athlete is unconscious place their arms across their chest
15. Attach the straps, ensuring the shoulder straps are in a 'seat belt' position, and a strap is placed over the hips/thigh and the lower leg
16. Straps should be tightened, and excess length tucked away
17. Apply the head blocks, ensuring MILS is maintained until the head straps are applied
18. Lift the athlete with one person at the head and two either side of the board, walking in the direction of their feet

Clearing the Neck

If the athlete is alert and shows no sign of concussion you may be able to clear their neck from injury following the Canadian C-Spine Rules [16]. If at any point in this process the athlete is unable to perform an instructed movement or they experience pain they should be immobilised and extracted via spinal board.

1. Assume the MILS position
2. Maintaining MILS, palpate the cervical spine, checking for pain or neural symptoms at each level
3. Instruct the athlete that you are going to ask them to perform movements for you, if they feel any pain or discomfort at any point, they should stop immediately
4. Maintaining MILS ask the athlete to rotate their head to look over their shoulder
5. Return to neutral and repeat for the other side
6. Maintaining MILS ask the athlete to extend their neck, return to neutral followed by neck flexion
7. Maintaining the MILS position passively perform neck rotation, extension and flexion
8. If no pain or neural symptoms have been provoked the athlete may slowly sit up

Concussion Assessment and Management

Sport Related Concussion is defined as a traumatic brain injury induced by biomechanical forces, caused either through a direct blow to the head or through the transmission of force to the head from an indirect blow to another part of the body [17]. While a concussion can only be diagnosed by a qualified medical practitioner it is essential any therapist can recognise a concussive event, and the subsequent onset of neurological impairment occurring either immediately or within the following hours [17]. Any individual suspected of suffering from concussion should be removed from play immediately.

Signs and Symptoms

Visible

- Loss of consciousness
- Tonic posturing
- Ataxia
- Confusion or vacant look
- Observable injury

Symptoms

- Headache
- Dizziness
- Vision problems
- Sensitivity to light or noise
- Nausea
- Fatigue

On Pitch Assessment

A short assessment on pitch can be used to recognise a potential concussion, on pitch assessment may include:

Maddock's questions [18]

- What venue are we at today?
- Which half is it now?
- Who scored last in this match?
- What team did we play last game?
- Did your team win last game?

Cervical Spine Assessment

- Pain free in resting
- Full active range of motion
- Normal strength and sensation of limbs

Balance Assessment

- Ask the athlete to stand on one leg for 20–30 seconds

Off Pitch Assessment

Following the removal from play a more comprehensive assessment can be made. Simple to use assessment tools are available, including the Sport Concussion Assessment Tool 5 (SCAT5) [19], which assesses the individual's symptoms, orientation, immediate memory, concentration, neural status, balance and delayed recall memory.

It is important for all therapists to understand that this test is not a diagnosis of concussion, it is a recognition tool, and the results will vary between individuals. For effective use individuals should completed baseline testing before being allowed to participate in contact and should not be allowed to return until they return to their baseline scores.

Post-concussion syndrome is a condition occurring when an individual presents with non-resolving symptoms, for longer than the usual recovery time of 10–14 days for adults or 4 weeks for children [19]. These individuals should be referred to an appropriate medical practitioner for assessment.

Glasgow Coma Scale

For a player that has been removed from the field of play via spinal board, a more comprehensive neurological disability assessment may be completed using the Glasgow Coma Scale (Table 4.1).

TABLE 4.1 Glasgow Coma Scale, adapted from Concussion In Sport Group recommendations [19]

Behaviour	Response	Score
Eye opening response	Spontaneously	4
	To speech	3
	To pain	2
	No response	1
Best verbal response	Orientated – time, location, person	5
	Confused	4
	Inappropriate words	3
	Incomprehensible	2
	No response	1
Best motor response	Obeys commands	6
	Responds to localised pain	5
	Flexion withdrawal from pain	4
	Abnormal flexion	3
	Abnormal extension	2
	No response	1

Return to Play Guidelines

Return to play timelines should be guided by the individual's symptoms. Sport regulation bodies may set out their own specific guidelines, many of which will include an initial 2-week rest period; however, the general Concussion In Sport Group recommendations [19] are the following (Table 4.2):

TABLE 4.2 Return to Play Guidelines, adapted from Concussion In Sport Group recommendations [19]

Initial rest period, both cognitive and physical, for 24–48 hours allowing symptoms to settle			
Stage 1	Symptom limited activities	Normal daily activities can be resumed as symptoms allow	Minimum 24 hours
Stage 2	Light aerobic activity	Slow to medium paced cardio, e.g. bike or slow jog. No resistance training	between stages
Stage 3	Sport specific activities	Introduction of running drills, no head impact	
Stage 4	Non-contact training	Introduction of sport specific drills, e.g. passing, agility. Introduction of resistance training	
Stage 5	Full training	Return to full team training. ★Must be approved by a suitably qualified medical practitioner★	
Stage 6	Return to sport	Return to competition	

Cryotherapy

Physiological Response

Cryotherapy is the application of cold in order to assist muscle recovery and control inflammation following injury or exercise. There are various forms of cryotherapy including ice, chemical cold packs, cold water immersion, whole body immersion, cryotherapy chambers and cold sprays. On application of cold therapy, the body commonly undergoes the Hunting Response of initial vasoconstriction is followed by alternating vasodilation and vasoconstriction [20]. However, there is also the possibility that the body will react with constant vasoconstriction, where the diameter remains the same or a process of slow steady re-warming [20]. The effectiveness of these therapies depends on its ability to reduce the temperature of the tissues as well as the depth of cooling achieved [21].

Ice and chemical cold packs are commonly used in the treatment of acute injuries, causing vasoconstriction, reducing blood flow to the area, reducing swelling, reducing cell metabolism as well as providing an analgesic effect [21]. Therapies such as cold water immersion, whole body immersion either in water or within cryotherapy chambers can be used to aid in the recovery of muscles following exercise by reducing inflammation, providing pain relief, reducing blood flow and tissue metabolism leading to increased removal of muscle metabolites as well as hormone alterations [22]. Theoretically these effects lead to an enhanced muscle recovery process. Whilst these methods are commonly employed within professional sporting environments, the overall effectiveness of them to aid muscle recovery is still in contention [23].

Guidelines for Use

Acute Injury

Apply ice to the area for 10–20 minutes, do not allow ice to remain on the area for greater than 30 minutes. Ice can be reapplied after a period of removal; this should be guided by comfort levels of the individual [21].

Cold Water Immersion for Recovery

Ice bath of 11–15° for a period of 11–15 minutes [24], depth of the water will depend on the targeted area.

Cryotherapy Chambers for Recovery

Duration and temperature will depend on the facilities used, generally, whole body cryotherapy is normally performed at temperatures between 110° and140° for 2 minutes [25].

Contraindications

- Raynaud's disease
- Circulatory insufficiency or disorders
- Cold hypersensitivity
- Recent MI (heart attack)
- Lower back or spinal related pain

Cautions

- Ice burns
- Anaesthesia (loss of sensation)
- Superficial nerve damage

Thermotherapy

Physiological Response

Thermotherapy is the application of heat, generally used in order to relieve pain and to facilitate the healing process. Once past the acute stages (48–72 hours) of injury the increase in blood flow to the area provided by heat can facilitate the healing process, allowing an increase in the phagocytes and nutrients delivered to the area, as well as efficient waste removal.

Heat has also been proposed to reduce pain due to the pain gate mechanism [26], in which the stimulation of cutaneous A_β nerve fibres results in a blocking effect, preventing A^δ and C nerve fibres pain signals being transmitted to the brain.

Thermotherapy has been shown to be effective in relieving lower back pain and should be used in preference of ice for all back pain as ice can increase the neurological sensitivity.

Heat can be applied through the use of hot water bottles, gel hot packs or heat packs.

Guidelines for Use

Apply heat to the area of pain for 10–20 minutes as required. Monitor the area throughout treatment for the prevention of burns.

Contraindications

- Acute injury
- Circulatory insufficiency or disorders
- Heat hypersensitivity
- Burns
- Anaesthesia (loss of sensation)

Contrast Water Immersion

Physiological Response

Contrast water immersion, also known as contrast bathing, is the application of alternating hot and cold water in order to relieve pain and assist with recovery, through alternate vasoconstriction and vasodilation, creating a 'pump' action [27]. Whilst contrast water immersion has been shown to have a an increased effect on muscle recovery compared to cold water immersion [28], it should not be used in the acute stages of injury.

Guidelines for Use

- Temperature: cold water 10°–12°, warm water 38°–42°
- Time: 60–90 seconds
- Cycles: 5–7 [28–29]

Contraindications

- Acute injury
- Raynaud's disease
- Circulatory insufficiency or disorders
- Recent MI (heart attack)

Over-Training Syndrome

Increases in load and training are commonly used within training programmes in order to improve an individual's performance. In order to obtain these performance increases consideration must be given to the rest periods allowed and periodisation of the programme [30]. Without these considerations there is a risk that Over-Reaching (OR) or Over-Training Syndrome (OTS) may develop.

Over-reaching is the accumulation of stress over a short period of time which results in performance deficits for days up to weeks [31]. This may occur as either functional or Non-Functional Over-Reaching. Functional Over-Reaching occurs when an individual undergoes a short increase in load, followed by a short recovery period of days to weeks, leading to an overall increase in performance [31]. Non-Functional Over-Reaching occurs when the balance of rest and load is disturbed, leading to longer performance deficits of weeks to months [31].

Over-Training Syndrome occurs when there is a long-term accumulation of stress, leading to long-term performance deficits, which may also be accompanied by psychological disturbances, illness, inadequate nutrition, hormonal disturbances or sleep disorders [30–31]. These various symptoms may also be apparent within Non-Functional Over-Reaching, therefore making a clinical distinction between the two may be difficult. Treatment for Non-Functional Over-Reaching and Over-Training Syndrome involves adequate rest [32].

Whilst prevention strategies involve monitoring an individual's load through Rate of Perceived Exertion [30] as well as monitoring the individuals psychological state through use of Profile of Mood States questionnaires such as the Recovery-Stress Questionnaire for Athletes [30, 33]. Hormonal testing may be valuable in identifying physiological stress, however the equipment and training for this testing is not always available to the therapist. Arguably the most important factor for prevention of Over-Training Syndrome is education of the individual to ensure they understand the risk factors and ensure all precautions are being taken to reduce the risk of Over-Training Syndrome or Non-Functional Over-Reaching [30–31, 34].

Nutrition for Exercise and Injury Recovery

An individual's nutritional intake is believed to have an impact on their performance, recovery post exercise, as well as on their recovery from injury. This includes the intake of macronutrients such as fats, proteins and carbohydrates as well as micronutrients such as vitamins and minerals. With all nutritional recommendations, it can be suggested that a food first approach is employed, promoting the intake of nutrients through a balanced diet rather than via supplements, where possible [35]. In the event that supplements are required it is essential to ensure they comply with any anti-doping regulations.

Performance

Prior and during any event it is essential that athletes have adequate glycogen stores, for the amount of energy to be used during the event, in order to prevent fatigue or reduce performance [36]. Similarly, glycogen stores must be replenished post event for recovery. Exact requirements will vary between individuals, so it is important the athlete knows what works for them. General recommendations set by American College of Sports Medicine for guaranteeing adequate glycogen stores are [36]:

Pre-Match

- In the 24 hours prior to the event the athletes reduce activity or energy expenditure and increases their carbohydrate intake to 7–12g/kg; this is known as carbohydrate loading
- For endurance sports (longer than 90 minutes of activity) this may be increased to 10–12g/kg over 36–48-hour period, allowing adequate glycogen stores
- Pre-event snacks or meals within 1–4 hours of activity should contain 1–4g/kg of carbohydrates
- In the 24 hours prior to the event foods should have a low fat and fibre content with a moderate protein content to allow gastrointestinal balance

During Match

See Hydration.

Post-Match

- Generally, glycogen stores can be replenished over the following hours through the intake of a balance diet
- In situations where an athlete has less than 8 hours before the next event, 1–1.2g/kg/h of carbohydrates should be ingested for the first 4–6 hours
- Protein has been shown to not only assist recovery, it may also enhance the recovery of glycogen stores; 20–30g of protein is recommended for recovery.

Injury Recovery

An injured athlete will normally reduce their daily calorie intake in order to balance their energy demands with their reduction in activity caused by injury. However, during this time the athlete's body will require energy in order to recover, in addition to which they may be training at a reduced load, therefore it is essential that intake is not decreased excessively as this will hinder their recovery process. Specific nutrients have been suggested as being beneficial for recovery depending on the structure that is injured [35].

Muscle Injuries

Due to the mechanism of muscle injuries being either traumatic or due to a rapid increase in muscle length, there is no real suggestion that nutrition may be able to play a role in the prevention of injury. However, protein supplements are commonly used for recovery post exercise, specifically to facilitate an increase in lean muscle mass [37]. Following an injury there may be a requirement for immobilisation which is likely to result in the loss of lean muscle mass, in addition to which the athlete is likely to reduce their overall calorie intake to match the reduction in energy output. It is suggested that the subsequent loss of lean muscle mass may be limited during this time through an increase of protein intake to 2.3g/kg [35]. Various other nutrients have been suggested to affect the inflammatory response to muscle injuries and to reduce the amount of atrophy during injury, including Vitamin D, Polyphenols and Creatine [35].

Bone Injuries

Traumatic bone injuries cannot be prevented through diet; however, overuse bone injuries and the promotion of bone healing for all injuries may be influence by nutritional intake. Insufficient energy intake has been linked to the occurrence of overuse bone injuries such as stress fractures. Whilst this is commonly associated with females and the Female Athlete Triad, energy deficiency may also result in bone overuse injuries within the male population [38]. It is suggested that an energy intake of 45 kcal·kg LBM−1·day−1 can reduce the risk of stress fractures occurring, although this may need further consideration within endurance sports [35]. It is widely known that the intake of calcium is essential for bone health and growth, in addition to which Vitamin D is required for calcium absorption [39]. Whilst there is little research on the effect of calcium and Vitamin D on bone healing directly, they are an important nutritional requirement to consider in an athlete with bone stress injuries and may be beneficial in facilitating bone healing [39]. Overall a wide range of macronutrients and micronutrients are essential for bone health and growth; however, energy deficiency, along with calcium and Vitamin D intake, are the most influential factors to consider during injury recovery [39].

Tendon and Ligament Injuries

Whilst there is no direct link between nutrition and tendon or ligament healing, the intake of various nutrients is essential for collagen synthesis, which is in turn vital to the healing of these tissues. Therefore, nutritional intake can indirectly influence tendon and ligament healing by ensuring the adequate collagen synthesis. Vitamin C and copper are essential in the production of collagen and should be included in a balanced daily diet as per daily intake recommendations [40].

There is no evidence to suggest that increased intake of Vitamin C or copper increases the healing rate, and therefore the use of supplements in facilitating healing would only be beneficial in individuals suffering from a specific deficiency [35]. In addition to this, other nutrients such as gelatine and glycine potentially improve collagen synthesis and may be useful during injury recovery [35].

Hydration

Sweat during exercise is the body's primary way of reducing body temperature; this leads to a loss in water and electrolytes which may result in dehydration and hyponatremia. In turn dehydration and hyponatremia can have various detrimental effects on an athlete's performance such as increased fatigue, muscle cramping and an increase in cardiovascular strain as well as athlete perceived exertion [41–42]. Conversely, hyper-hydration has also been suggested to have a negative impact on performance as it may lead to a reduction in blood sodium levels resulting in hyponatremia [41]. Therefore, ensuring adequate hydration is essential for athlete performance, and should be taken into consideration pre, during and post-training or match.

An individual's hydration needs can vary widely based on various factors such as diet, age, sex, environment, duration of exercise, body weight, heat acclimatisation and medications [41]. Therefore, hydration plans should ideally be customised to suit the individual; however, below sets out a general guide to ensure adequate hydration during exercise.

Pre-Match

- Athletes should consume approximately 500mLs, or 3–5mL per kg body weight, 1–2 hours prior to activity
- Water loss during activity can easily be monitored through body weight. In order to do this the athlete should be weighed pre-match with an empty bladder and in the same minimal clothing as they will be weighed post-match, e.g. playing kit

During Match

- Drink small amounts of water regularly throughout exercise to equal the amount of sweat lost
- Depending on the duration an intensity of the activity, carbohydrate drinks or other supplements may be used to help maintain energy, electrolyte balance and hydration during exercise [43]
- Carbohydrate intake during endurance sports of 30–60g/h or 90g/h in ultra-endurance is recommended [36]

Post-Match

- Athletes should be weighed in same clothing as pre-match. To calculate water loss, you can use the following formula:

    Pre-weight (kg) − Post-weight (kg) × 1.5 = Litres of water to be consumed

- Athletes with significant water loss should consume 500 ml immediately, with the remainder volume to be consumed over the following hours
- Food intake can assist in re-establishing electrolyte and fluid balances post exercise

Using Mental Skills in Injury Rehabilitation

Impact of Injuries

There has long been an awareness of the psychological impact injuries have on athletes [44–46], yet often this can be overlooked during the rehabilitation process. The vast majority of emphasis is often placed on the physiological impact of the injury yet being able to manage the psychological impact is key. The rehabilitation process itself is largely associated with negative emotions [47]. The ability to use mental skills during the injury rehabilitation process has widely been documented as being beneficial to athletes [48], in order to manage their psychological state.

Some of the core physiological and psychological implications of sport injury are highlighted below [49]:

- Perceived lack of progress
- Inability to partake in training and competition
- Reduction in fitness
- Comparison with uninjured athletes
- The timing of rehabilitation relative to competition
- Perceived lack of rehabilitation progression

Athletes are broadly aware, at the professional level at least, of at least one mental skill (96%), but only 13% of the sample indicated they'd used mental skills during an injury rehabilitation process [50]. This relatively low percentage is also supported by the findings (27%) of Arvinen-Burrow and colleagues [51]. Whilst athletes broadly use a range of mental skills during training and competition, their use during an injury rehabilitation process is less prominent.

The role of support teams during rehabilitation is also key. Physiotherapists' awareness around managing the psychological impact of injuries is well documented, with elements of their training being centred around it [52–53]. Apart from physiotherapists and athletic trainers, the availability of appropriately trained practitioners (sport psychologists) to oversee the provision of a mental skills training programme is often limited [54–55]. Additionally, it's pivotal for the mental skills component of the programme to be fully integrated into the rehabilitation process [45], and not to be viewed as a programme in its own right.

Increasing confidence is pivotal during the rehabilitation process [56]. If we examine Bandura's self-efficacy theory [57], there are four elements which influence the development of self-efficacy, which is situation specific self-confidence. These are past performance, vicarious experience, verbal feedback, and physiological states [58]. Creating a roadmap for athletes to negotiate, grow their confidence along the way can have a substantial impact on the rehabilitation process. Key to this is past performance, which is the most important predictor of subsequent self-efficacy [58]. Hence giving athletes the chance to experience early success within the programme will make them more confident overall.

A goal-setting framework can provide excellent structure and opportunities to review progress of the process. Goals have widely been used to build motivation [59–61], which is key for injured athletes [51].

Lastly, visualisation is widely documented in having a positive impact on athletes recovering from injury [62–63]. Positive effects associated with the use of visualisation are greater focus, sustained motivation, increased confidence and a reduction in anxiety.

Recommendations

Goals – Using process goals throughout the rehabilitation process, evaluating and reflecting on them with a person overseeing it. Process goals will be centred within the injured athlete's control, primarily assist in supporting motivation and create an unobtrusive and brutal measurement element. Using fixed outcome and performance goals could in situations create a lot of pressure and be quite damaging, particularly if these are not achieved. Being able to be ready to participate in an important fixture, reach a target body weight, or achieve a particular number in the gym can further increase anxiety and peer comparison, thus isn't preferred, at least in the early stages. Goals often work in conjunction with self-confidence [61]. Establishing significant levels of motivation and confidence (see below) are a good platform to then set performance related goals and prepare to fully immerse themselves back into their athletic programme.

Self-confidence – Building confidence within the injured athlete, in order for them to be more comfortable with the process they are in, can be further supported in a number of ways. From the literature above [56, 58], consider the following:

- Giving the athlete an opportunity for achievement; past performance is the most significant predictor of self-efficacy. Using a programme of process goals (see above) and measuring progress within them will start to build the athlete's self-efficacy.
- Peer/coach feedback is also pivotal in helping the athlete feel more confident in what they are doing. The person giving them the positive feedback is also significant. Ideally, they will be someone with a high degree of expertise in the athlete's environment and/or their medical condition. Examples of these could be the head coach, athletic director, doctor or physiotherapist. Having consistent input from a key person will help grow the athlete's confidence, and further validate their sense of achievement.
- Also, along the lines of the verbal persuasion element of self-efficacy, utilising a self-talk programme will help athletes recognise their own achievements, and give themselves feedback. Whilst feedback from others is powerful, the athlete should not become reliant on it, hence self-talk lends itself well to supporting their sense of self-efficacy within the rehabilitation process.
- Utilising visualisation can be beneficial for injured athletes, seeing as it requires no physical movement. Visualising achievement of their process goals, the injury healing, feeling well, being physically fit, confident and happy is key, and could initially be preferred to outcome visualisation.
- Lastly, integrating mental skills practice within the rehabilitation programme is pivotal, rather than it being perceived as a separate entity. It being supported by an appropriately trained practitioner (sport psychologist) is particularly important, in order for them to supervise the athlete and offer appropriate expertise. While not every athlete may have access to a sport psychologist, where possible, athletes, sports teams and governing bodies should seek appropriate support.

References

1. Perrin, D. H. (2012). *Athletic taping and bracing*. Champaign, IL: Human Kinetics.
2. MacDonald, R. (2009) *Pocketbook of taping techniques*. London: Churchill Livingstone.
3. McConnell J. (1986). The management of chondromalacia patellae: a long term solution. *The Australian journal of physiotherapy, 32*(4), 215–223. https://doi.org/10.1016/S0004-9514(14)60654-1

4. Williams, S., Whatman, C., Hume, P. A., & Sheerin, K. (2012). Kinesio taping in treatment and prevention of sports injuries: a meta-analysis of the evidence for its effectiveness. *Sports medicine, 42*(2), 153–164. https://doi.org/10.2165/11594960-000000000-00000

5. Hsu, Y. H., Chen, W. Y., Lin, H. C., Wang, W. T., & Shih, Y. F. (2009). The effects of taping on scapular kinematics and muscle performance in baseball players with shoulder impingement syndrome. *Journal of electromyography and kinesiology: official journal of the International Society of Electrophysiological Kinesiology, 19*(6), 1092–1099. https://doi.org/10.1016/j.jelekin.2008.11.003

6. Guner, S., Alsancak, S., & Koz, M. (2015). Effect of two different kinesio taping techniques on knee kinematics and kinetics in young females. *Journal of physical therapy science, 27*(10), 3093–3096. https://doi.org/10.1589/jpts.27.3093

7. Thedon, T., Mandrick, K., Foissac, M., Mottet, D., & Perrey, S. (2011). Degraded postural performance after muscle fatigue can be compensated by skin stimulation. *Gait & posture, 33*(4), 686–689. https://doi.org/10.1016/j.gaitpost.2011.02.027

8. Craighead, D., Shank, S., Volz, K. and Alexander, L. (2017). Kinesiology tape modestly increase skin blood flow regardless of tape application technique. *Journal of performance health research, 1*(1), 72–78.

9. Driscoll, P., & Skinner, D. (1990). ABC of major trauma. Initial assessment and management – I: primary survey. *BMJ, 300*(6734), 1265–1267. https://doi.org/10.1136/bmj.300.6734.1265

10. Driscoll, P., & Skinner, D. (1990). ABC of major trauma. Initial assessment and management – II: secondary survey [published correction appears in *BMJ* 1990 16 June, *300*(6739), 1575]. *BMJ, 300*(6735), 1329–1333. doi:10.1136/bmj.300.6735.1329

11. World Health Organisation. (2020). *The ABCDE and sample history approach.* https://www.who.int/emergencycare/publications/BEC_ABCDE_Approach_2018a.pdf

12. Fitzpatrick, D., McKenna, M., Duncan, E. A. S., Laird, C., Lyon, R. & Corfield, A. (2018). Critcomms: a national cross-sectional questionnaire based study to investigate prehospital handover practices between ambulance clinicians and specialist prehospital teams in Scotland. *Scand J trauma resusc emerg med, 26*(1), 45. https://doi.org/10.1186/s13049-018-0512-3

13. Payne, R., Kinmont, J. C., & Moalypour, S. M. (2004). Initial management of closed fracture-dislocations of the ankle. *Annals of the Royal College of Surgeons of England, 86*(3), 177–181. https://doi.org/10.1308/003588404323043300

14. Lee, C., & Porter, K. M. (2005). Prehospital management of lower limb fractures. *Emergency medicine journal, 22*(9), 660–663. https://doi.org/10.1136/emj.2005.024489

15. Joint Royal Colleges Ambulance Liaison Committee. (2006). *UK Ambulance Service Clinical Practice Guidelines (2006).* https://aace.org.uk/wp-content/uploads/2017/12/JRCALC_clinical_guidelines_2006.pdf

16. Stiell, I. G., Wells, G. A., Vandemheen, K. L., Clement, C. M., Lesiuk, H., De Maio, V. J., Laupacis, A., Schull, M., McKnight, R. D., Verbeek, R., Brison, R., Cass, D., Dreyer, J., Eisenhauer, M. A., Greenberg, G. H., MacPhail, I., Morrison, L., Reardon, M., & Worthington, J. (2001). The Canadian C-spine rule for radiography in alert and stable trauma patients. *JAMA, 286*(15), 1841–1848. https://doi.org/10.1001/jama.286.15.1841

17. McCrory, P., Feddermann-Demont, N., Dvořák, J., Cassidy, J. D., McIntosh, A., Vos, P. E., Echemendia, R. J., Meeuwisse, W., & Tarnutzer, A. A. (2017). What is the definition of sports-related concussion: a systematic review. *British journal of sports medicine, 51*(11), 877–887. https://doi.org/10.1136/bjsports-2016-097393

18. Maddocks, D. L., Dicker, G. D., & Saling, M. M. (1995). The assessment of orientation following concussion in athletes. *Clinical journal of sport medicine: official journal of the Canadian Academy of Sport Medicine, 5*(1), 32–35. https://doi.org/10.1097/00042752-199501000-00006

19. McCrory, P., Meeuwisse, W., Dvořák, J., Aubry, M., Bailes, J., Broglio, S., Cantu, R. C., Cassidy, D., Echemendia, R. J., Castellani, R. J., Davis, G. A., Ellenbogen, R., Emery, C., Engebretsen, L., Feddermann-Demont, N., Giza, C. C., Guskiewicz, K. M., Herring, S., Iverson, G. L., Johnston, K. M., & Vos, P. E. (2017). Consensus statement on concussion in sport – the 5th international conference on concussion in sport held in Berlin, October 2016. *British journal of sports medicine, 51*(11), 838–847. https://doi.org/10.1136/bjsports-2017-097699

20. Daanen, H. A. (2003). Finger cold-induced vasodilation: a review. *European journal of applied physiology,* *89*(5), 411–426. https://doi.org/10.1007/s00421-003-0818-2

21. Association of Chartered Physiotherapists in Sports and Exercises Medicine. (2010). *Acute management of soft tissue injuries.* https://www.physiosinsport.org/media/wysiwyg/ACPSM_Physio_Price_A4.pdf

22. Ihsan, M., Watson, G., & Abbiss, C. R. (2016). What are the physiological mechanisms for post-exercise cold water immersion in the recovery from prolonged endurance and intermittent exercise?. *Sports medicine, 46*(8), 1095–1109. https://doi.org/10.1007/s40279-016-0483-3

23. Holmes, M., & Willoughby, D. S., (2016) The effectiveness of whole body cryotherapy compared to cold water immersion: implications for sport and exercise recovery. *International journal of kinesiology and sports science, 4*(4), 32–39. doi:10.7575/aiac.ijkss.v.4n.4p.32.

24. Machado, A. F., Ferreira, P. H., Micheletti, J. K., de Almeida, A. C., Lemes, Í. R., Vanderlei, F. M., Netto Junior, J., & Pastre, C. M. (2016). Can water temperature and immersion time influence the effect of cold water immersion on muscle soreness? A systematic review and Meta-analysis. *Sports medicine, 46*(4), 503–514. https://doi.org/10.1007/s40279-015-0431-7

25. Banfi, G., Lombardi, G., Colombini, A., & Melegati, G. (2010). Whole-body cryotherapy in athletes. *Sports medicine, 40*(6), 509–517. https://doi.org/10.2165/11531940-000000000-00000

26. Melzack, R., & Wall, P. D. (1965). Pain mechanisms: a new theory. *Science, 150*(3699), 971–979. https://doi.org/10.1126/science.150.3699.971

27. Cochrane, D. (2004). Alternating hot and cold water immersion for athlete recovery: a review. *Physical therapy in sport, 5*(1), 26–32. https://doi.org/10.1016/j.ptsp.2003.10.002

28. Higgins, T. R., Heazlewood, I. T., & Climstein, M. (2011). A random control trial of contrast baths and ice baths for recovery during competition in U/20 rugby union. *Journal of strength and conditioning research, 25*(4), 1046–1051. https://doi.org/10.1519/JSC.0b013e3181cc269f

29. Pournot, H., Bieuzen, F., Duffield, R., Lepretre, P. M., Cozzolino, C., & Hausswirth, C. (2011). Short term effects of various water immersions on recovery from exhaustive intermittent exercise. *European journal of applied physiology, 111*(7), 1287–1295. https://doi.org/10.1007/s00421-010-1754-6

30. Kreher J. B. (2016). Diagnosis and prevention of overtraining syndrome: an opinion on education strategies. *Open access journal of sports medicine, 7*, 115–122. https://doi.org/10.2147/OAJSM.S91657

31. Meeusen, R., Duclos, M., Foster, C., Fry, A., Gleeson, M., Nieman, D., Raglin, J., Rietjens, G., Steinacker, J., Urhausen, A., European College of Sport Science, & American College of Sports Medicine (2013). Prevention, diagnosis, and treatment of the overtraining syndrome: joint consensus statement of the European College of Sport Science and the American College of Sports Medicine. *Medicine and science in sports and exercise, 45*(1), 186–205. https://doi.org/10.1249/MSS.0b013e318279a10a

32. Budgett, R. (1998). Fatigue and underperformance in athletes: the overtraining syndrome. *British journal of sports medicine, 32*(2), 107–110. https://doi.org/10.1136/bjsm.32.2.107

33. Kallus, K. W., & Kellmann, M. (2016). *The recovery-stress questionnaires : User manual.* Champaign, IL: Human Kinetics.

34. Budgett, R. (1990). Overtraining syndrome. *British journal of sports medicine, 24*(4), 231–236. https://doi.org/10.1136/bjsm.24.4.231

35. Close, G. L., Sale, C., Baar, K., & Bermon, S. (2019). Nutrition for the prevention and treatment of injuries in track and field athletes. *International journal of sport nutrition and exercise metabolism, 29*(2), 189–197. https://doi.org/10.1123/ijsnem.2018-0290

36. Thomas, D. T., Erdman, K. A., & Burke, L. M. (2016). American College of Sports Medicine joint position statement. Nutrition and athletic performance. *Medicine and science in sports and exercise, 48*(3), 543–568. https://doi.org/10.1249/MSS.0000000000000852

37. Morton, R. W., Murphy, K. T., McKellar, S. R., Schoenfeld, B. J., Henselmans, M., Helms, E., Aragon, A. A., Devries, M. C., Banfield, L., Krieger, J. W., & Phillips, S. M. (2018). A systematic review, meta-analysis and meta-regression of the effect of protein supplementation on resistance training-induced gains in muscle mass and strength in healthy adults. *British journal of sports medicine, 52*(6), 376–384. https://doi.org/10.1136/bjsports-2017-097608

38. Papageorgiou, M., Elliott-Sale, K. J., Parsons, A., Tang, J., Greeves, J. P., Fraser, W. D., & Sale, C. (2017). Effects of reduced energy availability on bone metabolism in women and men. *Bone, 105*, 191–199. https://doi.org/10.1016/j.bone.2017.08.019

39. Karpouzos, A., Diamantis, E., Farmaki, P., Savvanis, S., & Troupis, T. (2017). Nutritional aspects of bone health and fracture healing. *Journal of osteoporosis, 2017*, 4218472. https://doi.org/10.1155/2017/4218472

40. British Nutrition Foundation. (2019). *Nutrition requirements*. https://www.nutrition.org.uk/attachments/article/907/Nutrition%20Requirements_Revised%20August%202019.pdf

41. American College of Sports Medicine, Sawka, M. N., Burke, L. M., Eichner, E. R., Maughan, R. J., Montain, S. J., & Stachenfeld, N. S. (2007). American College of Sports Medicine position stand. Exercise and fluid replacement. *Medicine and science in sports and exercise, 39*(2), 377–390. https://doi.org/10.1249/mss.0b013e31802ca597

42. Bergeron, M. F. (2003). Heat cramps: fluid and electrolyte challenges during tennis in the heat. *Journal of science and medicine in sport, 6*(1), 19–27. https://doi.org/10.1016/s1440-2440(03)80005-1

43. Oliveira, C. C., Ferreira, D., Caetano, C., Granja, D., Pinto, R., Mendes, B., & Sousa, M. (2017). Nutrition and supplementation in soccer. *Sports, 5*(2), 28. https://doi.org/10.3390/sports5020028

44. Weiss, M. R., & Troxel, R. K. (1986). Psychology of the injured athlete. *Athletic Training*, 21, 104–109.

45. Brewer, B., Jeffers, K., Petitpas, A., & Van Raalte, J. (1994). Perceptions of psychological interventions in the context of sport injury rehabilitation. *The sport psychologist, 8*(2), 176–188. https://doi.org/10.1123/tsp.8.2.176

46. Wiese-bjornstal, D., Smith, A., Shaffer, S., & Morrey, M. (1998). An integrated model of response to sport injury: psychological and sociological dynamics. *Journal of applied sport psychology, 10*(1), 46–69. https://doi.org/10.1080/10413209808406377

47. Evans, L., Hardy, L., Mitchell, I., & Rees, T. (2008). The development of a measure of psychological responses to injury. *Journal of sport rehabilitation, 17*(1), 21–37. https://doi.org/10.1123/jsr.17.1.21

48. Hare, R., Evans, L., & Callow, N. (2008). Imagery use during rehabilitation from injury: a case study of an elite athlete. *The sport psychologist, 22*(4), 405–422. https://doi.org/10.1123/tsp.22.4.405

49. Wadey, R., Evans, L., Hanton, S., & Neil, R. (2012). An examination of hardiness throughout the sport-injury process: A qualitative follow-up study. *British journal of health psychology, 17*(4), 872–893. https://doi.org/10.1111/j.2044-8287.2012.02084.x

50. Keilani, M., Hasenöhrl, T., Gartner, I., Krall, C., Fürnhammer, J., Cenik, F., & Crevenna, R. (2016). Use of mental techniques for competition and recovery in professional athletes. *Wiener klinische Wochenschrift, 128*(9–10), 315–319. https://doi.org/10.1007/s00508-016-0969-x

51. Arvinen-Barrow, M., Clement, D., Hamson-Utley, J. J., Zakrajsek, R. A., Lee, S. M., Kamphoff, C., Lintunen, T., Hemmings, B., & Martin, S. B. (2015). Athletes' use of mental skills during sport injury rehabilitation. *Journal of sport rehabilitation, 24*(2), 189–197. https://doi.org/10.1123/jsr.2013-0148

52. Hemmings, B., & Povey, L. (2002). Views of chartered physiotherapists on the psychological content of their practice: a preliminary study in the United Kingdom. *British journal of sports medicine, 36*(1), 61–64. https://doi.org/10.1136/bjsm.36.1.61

53. Heaney, C., Green, A.. K., Rostron, C. L. & Walker, N. (2012). A qualitative and quantitative investigation of the psychology content of UK physiotherapy education programs. *Journal of physical therapy education, 26*(3), 24–56.

54. Shapiro, J. L. (2009). *An individualized multimodal mental skills intervention for college athletes undergoing injury rehabilitation*. Virginia University. https://researchrepository.wvu.edu/cgi/viewcontent.cgi?article=5567&context=etd

55. Shapiro, J. L., & Etzel, E. F. (2018). An individualized multimodal mental skills intervention for injured college athletes. *Journal of contemporary athletics, 12*(4), 237–252.

56. Podlog, L., Dimmock, J., & Miller, J. (2011). A review of return to sport concerns following injury rehabilitation: practitioner strategies for enhancing recovery outcomes. *Physical therapy in sport: official journal of the Association of Chartered Physiotherapists in Sports Medicine, 12*(1), 36–42. https://doi.org/10.1016/j.ptsp.2010.07.005

57. Bandura, A. (1997). *Self efficacy: The exercise of control*. New York: Freeman.

58. Feltz, D. L., Short, S. E., & Sullivan, P. J. (2008). *Self-efficacy in sport*. Champaign, IL: Human Kinetics.

59. Locke, E. A., & Latham, G. P. (1990). *A theory of goal setting & task performance*. Englewood Cliffs, NJ: Prentice-Hall.

60. Locke, E. A., & Latham, G. P. (2002). Building a practically useful theory of goal setting and task motivation. A 35-year odyssey. *The American psychologist, 57*(9), 705–717. https://doi.org/10.1037//0003-066x.57.9.705

61. Locke, E. A., & Latham, G. P. (2006). New directions in goal-setting theory. *Current directions in psychological science, 15*(5), 265–268.

62. Monsma, E., Mensch, J., & Farroll, J. (2009). Keeping your head in the game: sport-specific imagery and anxiety among injured athletes. *Journal of athletic training, 44*(4), 410–417. https://doi.org/10.4085/1062-6050-44.4.410

63. Durden, M., & Marty Durden, E. D. (2017). Utilizing imagery to enhance injury rehabilitation. *Sport journal, 1.*

5

INJURY TREATMENT MODALITIES

Konstantinos Papadopoulos

Regular participation in sport and exercise has positive physical, mental and social health enhancing properties. However, regular participation in sport and exercise can sometimes have a detrimental effect on health in the form of injury. The effects that such injuries have on an individual's health depend on the type of injury and can range from a short period of rest needed, to more profound resulting in athletes having to retire from their careers. Knowing precisely how this process works is vital in knowing when to apply the correct treatment modality. Too soon could be inhibitory in nature and may even cause more damage, too late and a poor and detrimental outcome may result.

Soft Tissue Therapy

Soft tissue therapy also known as sports massage, is the systematic, mechanical stimulation of the oft tissue of the body by means of rhythmical applied pressure and stretching for therapeutic purposes. It has had a long tradition of use in sport and is used before, during and after sport events. Sports massage has been suggested as a means to help prepare an athlete for competition, as a tool to enhance athletic performance, as a treatment approach to help the athlete recover after exercise or competition, and as a manual therapy intervention for sports-related musculo-skeletal injuries [1–2]. Frequent claims made in the sports literature for the benefits of massage include improved stretching of tendons and connective tissue and relief of muscle tension and spasm [3–5].

Sport massage techniques are quite similar to Swedish massage. The main difference between sports and classic massage is that they serve different purposes, so they are applied differently. For example, sports massage in most cases is applied with great pressure as, due to sports adjustments, the body of the athlete requires a more aggressive approach, while there are manipulations that are used almost exclusively in the recovery of sports injuries [6]. Sport massage can be used before, during and after athletic events.

The main sport massage techniques are:

1. Effleurage
2. Petrissage
3. Tapotement

4. Vibration
5. Transverse friction

Effleurage

Every massage begins and ends with effleurage (Figure 5.1). The main purpose of this technique is for the therapist to apply the emollient, to evaluate the area and the psychological mood of the patient. The pressure exerted varies and depends on the purpose of the application. In case the goal is to reduce muscle tone, the pressure applied is mild, while in case the goal is to reduce swelling, the pressure applied is greater. This technique increases lymphatic flow and circulation [1].

Petrissage

The petrissage technique also known as kneading is used to reduce muscle tone, increase blood flow perspiration and dissolve adhesions locally, but also to increase the elasticity of the connective and muscle tissues (Figure 5.2). Kneading is performed on small and large surfaces and the way they are applied has several variations [2].

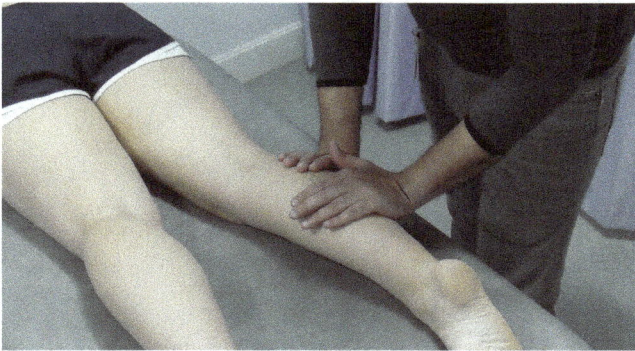

FIGURE 5.1   The effleurage technique.

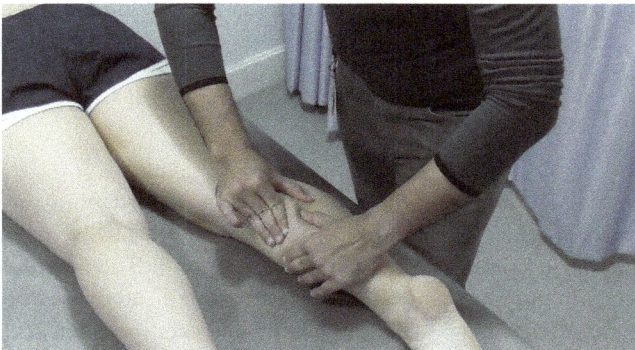

FIGURE 5.2   The petrissage technique.

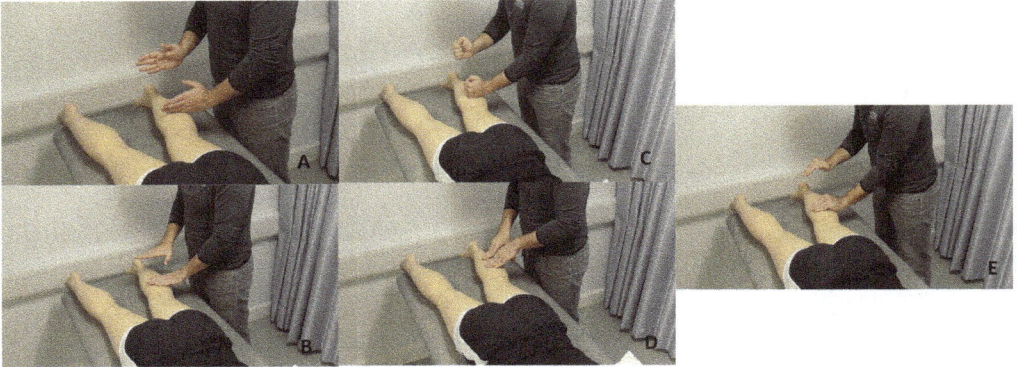

FIGURE 5.3   The tapotement techniques.

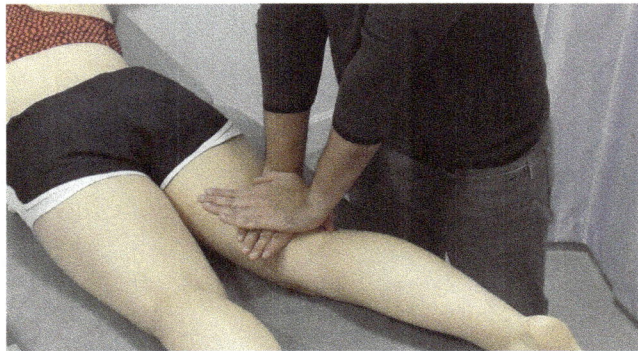

FIGURE 5.4   The vibration technique.

Tapotement

This technique uses a variety of percussive or beating techniques. Fingers, cupped hands or loosely held fists or the edge of the hand are used to apply rhythmical percussion strokes. The most common techniques are the A) hacking, B) slapping, C) beating, D) tapping and E) cupping (Figure 5.3). Tapotement is usually performed alternating hands and maintaining a fast pace of between four to ten strikes per second. Sixty seconds tends to be the minimum threshold where tapotement's effects kick in. It is also the most frequently used technique to energise the muscles and the nervous system in pre-event sports massage [1].

Vibrations

This technique, involves continuous oscillating movements applied from the therapist's palmar surface and aim to relax and increase blood flow. Static vibrations involve using therapist's whole hand or part the hand to apply continuous contact with the client's body without sliding over the client's skin. Running vibrations involves the therapist's whole hand or part of the hand to apply continuous contact with the client's body with a slight glide over the client's skin. The tension can be mild to intense (Figure 5.4). The vibration is created by the arms of the therapist and is transmitted to the tissues through the therapist's hands [2].

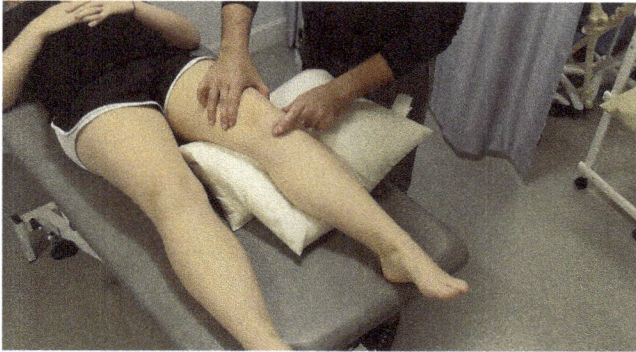

FIGURE 5.5   The transverse friction technique.

Transverse Friction

Transverse friction massage (also known as cross-friction and cross-fibre massage) is a specific massage technique developed by Cyriax. The main goal of this technique is to prevent the formation of adhesions at the initial stages of an injury and to release them when they have already been created in cases of poor rehabilitation. The main difference from the classic massage manipulations is that the transverse friction technique is applied directly the injured tissue. It is mainly used on tendon or ligament injuries to help break down thickened, pain-producing scar tissue and has a transverse direction. For correct application, the therapist's fingers and the patient's skin must move as a unit, otherwise there is a risk of skin injury (Figure 5.5). The duration of the technique is 10 minutes every 48 hours.

Other Soft Tissue Techniques

Active Release Techniques

Active Release Techniques (ART) are a soft tissue method that focuses on relieving tissue tension via the removal of fibrosis/adhesions which can develop in tissues as a result of overload due to repetitive use [7]. The goal is to break down scar tissue and adhesions in order to optimise function in the body. The technique can be applied to both acute and chronic conditions involving the muscles, tendons, ligaments, nerves and fascia. ART has been reported to be both a diagnostic and a treatment technique, however, there is little scientific evidence regarding the effects of ART on various pathologies, with most of the available evidence being anecdotal and based on case reports. During treatment, the therapist applies compressive, tensile and shear forces to address the injury. Whilst the therapist applies deep tension, the patient is instructed to lengthen their muscles [8]. On average, soft tissue treatment requires 2–6 visits (each lasting about 15–30 minutes).

Ischemic Compression

A trigger point (TrP) is a hyperirritable spot, a palpable nodule in the taut bands of the skeletal muscles' fascia. Ischemic pressure inactivates pain trigger points through two main mechanisms: a) Ischemia followed by hyperemia and b) local and focused tissue stretching. Ischemic pressure will initially create a reduction in local blood supply, while after the pressure is removed there will be a hyperemia of the area which can help to remove the inflammation. In addition, the constant localised pressure on the trigger points will lead to a prolonged stretch that can release painful muscle knots and reduce pain. For the successful application of the ischemic pressure, the affected muscle must be in a position of moderate stretching, which will cause little or no pain. The patient is placed in a relaxed position and the pressure is applied with the thumb or other finger or even with the elbow. The pressure should cause pain at a level tolerated by the patient. Ischemic pressure can be maintained for 10–20 seconds up to one minute [9].

Sport massage can:

• Reduce muscle pain	• Increase blood flow
• Decrease neuromuscular excitability	• Increase venous return
• Stimulate circulation	• Delay muscle atrophy
• Facilitate healing	• Increase range of motion
• Restore joint mobility	• Reduce oedema
• Remove lactic acid	• Align collagen fibres of scar tissue
• Alleviate muscle cramps	

Contra-Indications for Soft Tissue Therapy

Below you can find the most common contra-indications for massage. It is worth saying that literature shows that there is no agreement between experts regarding the absolute and relative contra-indications [10].

• Arteriosclerosis	• Synovitis
• Deep Venous Thrombosis	• Abscesses
• Severe varicose veins	• Skin infections
• Acute phlebitis	• Cancers
• Cellulitis	• Damaged blood vessels/bleeding
• Fragile skin	• Skin connective tissue diseases
• Acute inflammatory conditions	[11]

Stretching

Flexibility is the ability of a joint or series of joints to move through an unrestricted, pain-free range of motion. Although flexibility varies widely from person to person, minimum ranges are necessary for maintaining joint and total body health. Flexibility varies widely from person to person and is influenced by an array of factors such as anatomical structure, genetics, body type, temperature, age, gender, history of injury and activity levels [12].

Stretching is called the elongation of a soft tissue through appropriate methods with the aim of increasing the range of motion. It is a popular and basic component of most sports training and practice. Stretching exercises are very often included in the programme of athletes, especially during warm-up and recovery, and are widely accepted as an important factor in preventing injuries and improving performance. Stretching can be beneficial but can also lead to injury or reduced performance of athletes if not properly implemented in terms of both time and performance [13].

Flexibility can be achieved through various ways of stretching exercises and other techniques. Evidence shows that physical performance in terms of maximal strength, number of repetitions and total volume are all affected differently by each form of stretching.

The Three Types of Stretching

Three muscle stretching techniques are frequently described in the literature: Static, Dynamic, and Pre-Contraction stretches (Figure 5.6). The traditional and most common type is **static** stretching, where a specific position is held with the muscle on tension to a point of a stretching sensation and repeated. This can be performed passively by a therapist, or actively by the subject. The greatest change in ROM with a static stretch occurs between 15 and 30 seconds. Most authors suggest that 10 to 30 seconds is sufficient for increasing flexibility [14]. In addition, no increase in muscle elongation occurs after 2 to 4 repetitions [15].

There are two types of **dynamic** stretching: active and ballistic stretching. Many people confuse active stretching with ballistic stretching. Active stretching generally involves moving a limb through its full range of motion to the end ranges and repeating several times. Active stretching helps restore dynamic function and neuromuscular control through repeating and practicing movement thus enhancing motor control. Active stretching is sometimes considered preferable to static stretching in the preparation for physical activity [17]. Ballistic stretching includes rapid, alternating movements or 'bouncing' at end-range of motion; however, because of increased risk for injury, ballistic stretching is no longer recommended.

Pre-contraction stretching involves a contraction of the muscle being stretched or its antagonist before stretching. The most common type of pre-contraction stretching is the proprioceptive neuromuscular facilitation (PNF) stretching (see Table 5.1). There are three different types of PNF stretching including 'contract-relax' (C-R), 'hold-relax' (H-R) and 'contract-relax agonist contract' (CRAC). These techniques are generally performed by having the patient or client contract the muscle being used during the technique at 75 to 100% of maximal contraction, holding for 10 seconds, and then relaxing. Resistance can be provided by the therapist, an elastic band or strap. There are also other types of pre-contraction stretching such as the 'post-isometric relaxation'. This type of technique uses a much smaller amount of muscle contraction (25%) followed by a stretch. Post-facilitation stretch (PFS) is a technique developed by Dr Vladimir Janda that involves

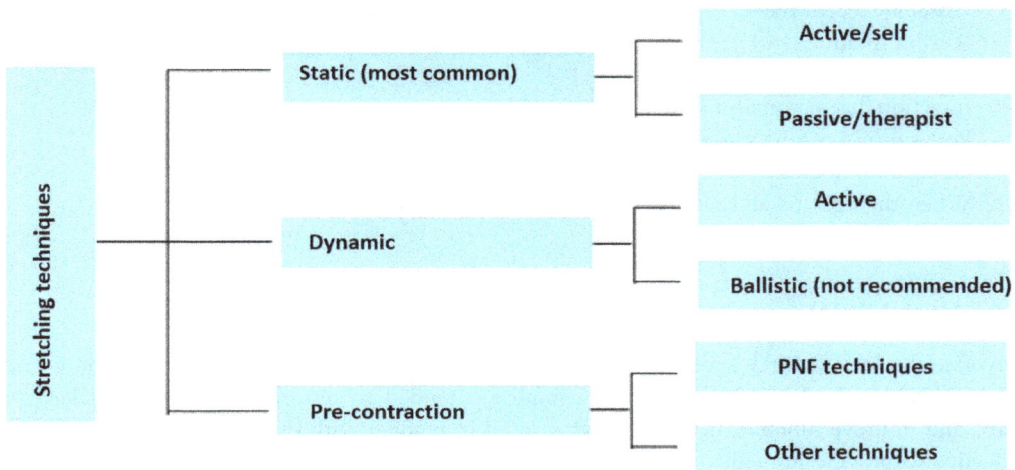

FIGURE 5.6   The stretching techniques (adopted from Page, 2012 'Current concepts in muscle stretching for exercise and rehabilitation' [16]).

TABLE 5.1 Types of PNF stretching

• Contract relax (CR)	Contraction of the muscle through its spiral-diagonal PNF pattern, followed by stretch
• Hold relax (HR)	Contraction of the muscle through the rotational component of the PNF pattern, followed by stretch
• Contract-relax agonist contract (CRAC)	Contraction of the muscle through its spiral-diagonal PNF pattern, followed by contraction of opposite muscle to stretch target muscle
	Adopted from Page (2012) [16]

a maximal contraction of the muscle at mid-range with a rapid movement to maximal length followed by a 15-second static stretch [18].

Both static and dynamic stretching techniques seem to have an effect on improving ROM acutely or over time with training. Previous research has shown that there is no improvement in performance when comparing static and dynamic stretching [19]. Although static stretching has been found to reduce strength and performance, dynamic stretching has been shown to improve dynamometer-measured power as well as jumping and running performance [20].

Indications for stretching:

- Muscle tightness or stiffness due to due to immobilisation, altered posture or injury
- Difference in length of antagonists and protagonists
- Restricted motion may lead to structural deformities that are otherwise preventable
- As a component of a total fitness or sport-specific conditioning programme designed to prevent or reduce the risk of musculoskeletal injuries

Contra-indications for stretching:

- Bony block on end of range on passive assessment
- Unstable/recent fracture
- Recent sprain
- Acute soft tissue injury
- Infection/haematoma in tissues
- Post-surgical repairs, e.g, skin grafts, tendon repair
- Hypermobility
- When the tight tissue can be used to stabilise a joint or make it functional
- Client refusal

Myofascial Release

Myofascial release (MFR) is a form of manual therapy that involves the application of a low load, long duration stretch to the myofascial complex, intended to restore optimal length, decrease pain, and improve function [21]. MFR when used in tandem with other treatment is said to be effective to provide immediate relief of pain and tissue tenderness [22]. Myofascial practitioners have hypothesised that fascial restrictions in one region of the body can cause undue stress in other regions of the body due to fascial continuity. This may result in stress on other regions or structures that are enveloped, divided, or supported by fascia [23]. It is believed that by stretching restricted fascia, myofascial release therapy is able to normalise the length and the sliding properties of myofascial tissues releasing also pressure from the pain-sensitive structures and restoring the mobility of the joints [24].

MFR generally involves slow, sustained pressure (120–300s) applied to restricted fascial layers either directly (direct MFR technique) or indirectly (indirect MFR technique). Direct MFR technique aims to work directly over the restricted fascia and practitioners use knuckles elbows or other tools to slowly sink into the fascia. The pressure applied is a few kilograms. Indirect MFR includes a gentle stretch guided along the path of least resistance until free movement is achieved. The pressure applied is a few grams of force, and the hands tend to follow the direction of fascial restrictions, hold the stretch, and allow the fascia to loosen itself [25]. A recent systematic review on the effectiveness of myofascial release in the treatment of chronic musculoskeletal pain showed that there is still not sufficient evidence to warrant this treatment in chronic musculoskeletal pain [26].

By extension, self-myofascial release (SMFR) is a type of MFR that is performed by the individual themselves rather than by a clinician, often using a tool. The most common tools used for SMFR are the foam roller and the roller massager [27–29]. Although SMFR appears to have various acute and chronic effects, there is currently no consensus regarding the exact mechanism or mechanisms by which SMFR leads to these effects. However, recent evidence shows that SMFR seems to lead to increased joint ROM acutely and does not impede athletic performance acutely. SMFR seems to alleviate DOMS acutely and may therefore be suitable for use by athletes or the general population for enhancing recovery from exercise, training sessions or competition [29].

Indications for MFR

MFR can be used to treat pain and increase mobility in patients with a wide range of conditions, including back pain, neck pain and fibromyalgia.

Athletes can also benefit. A number of sports injuries can be treated with MFR, including:

- Repetitive strain injuries, often seen in long distance runners
- Muscular imbalances, which lead to overuse in isolated joints and faulty movement patterns

Contra-Indications for MFR

Contra-indications for myofascial release (MFR) techniques include the following:

- Congenital connective tissue diseases or abnormalities (e.g. Ehlers-Danlos syndrome, a condition of hyperelasticity of connective tissue [abnormal soft tissue response])
- Friable or ruptured skin or subcutaneous soft tissues; acutely inflamed or infected soft tissues (i.e. unstable soft tissues)
- Hypersensitivity to touch (i.e. complex regional pain syndromes [patient intolerability])
- Muscle splinting or guarding due to underlying disease, fracture, or inflammation (i.e. abnormal response of soft tissues) (Adapted from Sheffinger [30])

Cupping

Cupping therapy is a technique that has been used since ancient times. Recently, there is growing evidence of its potential benefits in the treatment of pain-related diseases. Cupping is performed by applying cups of different size to selected skin points and creating suction by heat or mechanically by creating subatmospheric pressure [31]. The suction aims to increase the peripheral blood circulation and improve immunity.

Reported effects of cupping therapy include promotion of the skin's blood flow, change of the skin's biomechanical properties, increase pain thresholds, improve local anaerobic metabolism, inflammation decrease, and modulation of the cellular immune system [32–35]. Additionally, some authors suggest that cupping works in a similar way to acupuncture [36].

The cupping classification was recently updated in 2016 [37]. This updated classification categorised cupping therapy into six categories. The category includes dry, wet, massage and flash cupping.

With dry cupping, the cup is set in place for a set time, usually between 5 and 10 minutes. With wet cupping, cups are usually only in place for a few minutes before the practitioner removes the cup and makes a small incision to draw blood.

After the cups are removed, the practitioner may cover the previously cupped areas with ointment and bandages. This helps prevent infection. Any mild bruising or other marks usually go away within 10 days of the session.

Indications for cupping treatment:

- Health promotion, preventive and therapeutic purposes
- Low back pain
- Neck and shoulder pain
- Headache and migraine
- Facial paralysis
- Brachialgia
- Carpal tunnel syndrome
- Hypertension
- Diabetes mellitus
- Rheumatoid arthritis
- Asthma

Contra-indications for cupping treatment:

- Veins
- Arteries
- Nerves
- Skin inflammation
- Skin lesion
- Body orifices
- Eyes
- Lymph nodes
- Varicose veins
- Open wounds
- Bone fractures
- Sites of deep vein thrombosis

- Organ failure (renal failure, hepatic failure and heart failure)
- Cancer
- Pregnancy
- Anaemia [31]

Joint Mobilisation

Joint mobilisation techniques are one of the most widespread and internationally recognised therapeutic methods for the treatment of musculoskeletal disorders. In particular, they are considered one of the most conservative interventions for the assessment and treatment of musculoskeletal dysfunction in the joints and periarticular tissues [38].

Arhtrokinematics is the general term for the specific movements of joint surfaces. It is the 'motion you feel'. Arthrokinematic motion cannot occur independently or voluntarily and if restricted, can limit physiological movement. Unobservable articular accessory motion between adjacent joint surfaces: a) roll, b) glide and c) spin. These accessory motions take place with all active and passive movements and are necessary for full, pain-free range of motion [39].

Joint surfaces are defined as:

- Convex: male; rounded or arched
- Concave: female; hollowed or shallow

Rules of Motion

Choosing the direction of the mobilisation is integral to ensuring you are having the desired clinical outcome. This is why a knowledge of basic arthrokinematics is essential. There are two important rules to remember:

> When a convex surface (i.e Humeral Head) moves on a stable concave surface (i.e Glenoid Fossa) the sliding of the convex articulating surface occurs in the opposite direction to the motion of the bony lever (i.e the Humerus) [40]
>
> The opposite can be said for when a concave surface (i.e Tibia; tibiofemoral joint) is moving on a stable convex surface (i.e Femur) sliding occurs in the same direction of the bony level [40] (Figure 5.7)

An important part of arthrokinematics is the knowledge of loose and locked-packed position of the joints, which contributes to the appropriate assessment and treatment of joint problems through joint mobilisation. It is important that the initial position for accessory movements to be a position with high intra-articular mobility (loose-packed position).

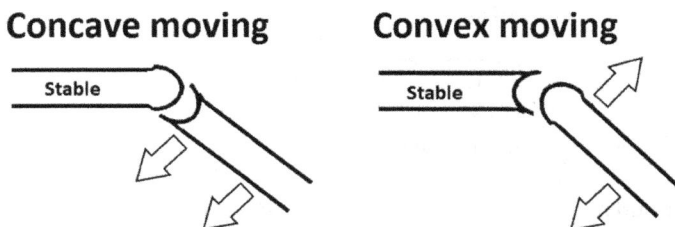

FIGURE 5.7 The convex–concave rule.

Another element of arthrokinematics that is very important for the treatment of the joint is the treatment plane. The treatment plane lies in the concave articular surface and is parallel to the joint surface and perpendicular to the axis in the convex surface. Determining the treatment plane is important for knowing the exact direction in which mobilisation should be performed. According to Kaltenborn [41] the treatment plane remains with the concave joint surface whether the moving joint partner is concave or convex.

Depending on the findings of the evaluation and the goal of the treatment, the rhythmic mobilisation is distinguished by four grades [42]:

• Grade I – small amplitude movement at the beginning of the available range of movement
• Grade II – large amplitude movement at within the available range of movement
• Grade III – large amplitude movement that moves into stiffness or muscle spasm
• Grade IV – small amplitude movement stretching into stiffness or muscle spasm

The grading scale has been separated into two due to their clinical indications:

Lower grades (I + II) are used to reduce pain and irritability.
Higher grades (III + IV) are used to stretch the joint capsule and passive tissues which support and stabilise the joint so increase range of movement.

The duration and frequency of the mobilisations depend on several factors such as: the joint, age, tissue damage etc. Although there are no suggested protocols to follow, the most common approach is 3 sets of one minute, 2–3 times per week.

Before You Attempt Joint Mobilisation

The **Direction** – of the mobilisation needs to be clinically reasoned by the therapist and needs to be appropriate for the diagnosis made. Not all directions will be effective for any dysfunction.

The **Desired Effect** – what effect of the mobilisation is the therapist wanting? Relieve pain or stretch stiffness?

The **Starting Position** – of the patient and the therapist to make the treatment effective and comfortable. This also involves thinking about how the forces from the therapist's hands will be placed to have a localised effect.

The **Method of Application** – The position, range, amplitude, rhythm and duration of the technique.

The **Expected Response** – Should the patient be pain-free, have an increased range or have reduced soreness?

How Might the Technique be **Progressed** – Duration, frequency or rhythm? [42]

Indications for joint mobilisation:

• Reduce pain (local or/and referred pain)
• Improve range of motion (ROM)
• Improve quality of joint movement and joint end-feel
• Improve tissue extensibility
• Improve joint nutrition

Contra-indications for joint mobilisation:

- Metastatic carcinoma
- Hemarthrosis
- Rheumatoid arthritis
- Ankylosing spondylitis
- Vascular disease, or acute infections related to the area to be treated
- Genetic disorders resulting in joint laxity such as Down syndrome
- Osteoporosis

Precautions for joint mobilisation:

- Pregnancy (due to the resultant increase in joint laxity)
- Hypermobility
- Spondylolisthesis
- Severe pain in the joint to
- Muscle guarding
- A fracture in the area
- Anticoagulant therapy
- Recent surgery in the area [38]

Hydrotherapy

Hydrotherapy is the use of water in the treatment of different conditions or recovery from hard training. It is a form of exercise in warm water and is a popular treatment in sport conditions [43]. The healing properties of the water have been known since Hippocratestimes, who practiced immersions in hot and cold water to treat various ailments such as muscle spasms and arthropathies. Since then, the therapeutic movement and exercise in the water has made a great progress. The reason is both the technological improvement and the evidence-based practice. Successful planning and implementation of a sports injury rehabilitation programme requires adequate knowledge of the natural principles and properties of water. The main properties of water are 1) buoyancy, 2) hydrostatic pressure, 3) water temperature and 4) water resistance.

Archimedes' principle, physical law of *buoyancy*, states that anybody completely or partially submerged in a fluid at rest is acted upon by an upward force, the magnitude of which is equal to the weight of the fluid displaced by the body. This upward impulse acts in the opposite direction from the gravitational pull and forces the body to float. In contrast to what happens on land, when exercising in water the movement is easier when performed on the surface of the water and it becomes more difficult towards the opposite direction [44]. The therapist may need the help of floating equipment during the rehabilitation of an athlete, such as foam water noodles, water dumbbells and boards, in order to increase the buoyancy of the body.

The direction of movement, the position of the body or limb in the water, the use of floating equipment, the lever of force, the speed of movement of the limb, together with the relative density of the water determine the type of muscle contraction and the type of the motion.

Due to **buoyancy**, exercise in water is safer than that in the land, especially in injuries where the injured limb is not allowed to be fully loaded. Overall, the more deeply the body is submerged, the less weight is borne by the lower extremities. The percentage of body weight, offloaded with

TABLE 5.2 Approximate percentage of body-mass offloaded with increasing immersion depth

Level of immersion	Standing male	Standing female	Slow paced ambulation male	Slow paced ambulation female
C7	8–10%	8–10%	25%	25%
Xyphoid process	35%	28%	25–50%	25–50%
ASIS	47%	54%	50–75%	50–75%

increasing immersion, depends on the relative density of the member relative to that of the water, and can vary either with the depth of immersion or with the use of equipment such as life jackets.

The percentages of bodyweight offloaded with increasing immersion depth is different for men and women and can be seen below (Table 5.2) [45].

Hydrostatic pressure is a fundamental property that is based on Pascal's principle and states that at a given depth, the pressure of the liquid is exerted equally on all surfaces of the submerged body [46]. The hydrostatic pressure place on the outside the body causes a decrease in blood pressure (BP) peripherally and an increase in the BP in and around the heart. This can cause potential problems for chronic heart failure (CHF) and coronary artery disease CAD) clients and needs to be taken into consideration. The greater the depth the greater the changes described above would be. However, when a client suffers from leg swelling then hydrotherapy can help if exercises are given well below the surface of the water where the increased pressure may be used [47].

The physiological effects of water therapy combine those brought by the hot water of the pool with those of the exercises. The extent of the effects varies with the temperature of the water, the length of the treatment and the type and severity of the exercise. Water has the ability to absorb/retain heat 1,000 times more than air and carries it 25 times faster, affecting the physiological function of all systems of the human body [48]. By immersing the body in warm water, lukewarm or cold water, changes are caused in the cardiovascular, respiratory, endocrine, urinary and musculoskeletal systems. **Water temperature** is an important factor in sport rehabilitation and must be adjusted according to the purpose and objectives of the program. For example, a temperature higher than 35°C can cause rapid fatigue, while exercise at a water temperature of 26°C can increase muscle tension or hypothermia. When the purpose is muscle relaxation, water temperature of 36–38°C is required, while for aerobic exercise the recommended temperature is 26–29°C. In addition to the water temperature, the air temperature of the room also plays an important role, which up to 30 degrees must be 1 degree higher than the water to prevent evaporation [44].

Water resistance is greater than that experienced during locomotion on dry land [49]. This greater resistance of water compared with that of air is due not only to its density, but also to its dynamic viscosity. The latter refers to the magnitude of the internal friction associated with a given fluid, in other words, its resistance to flow. When the whole body (or one of its extremities) moves through water it is subjected to three types of resistance: 1) shape resistance, 2) wave resistance, and 3) friction. Shape resistance is caused by the fact that movement through water produces an area of high pressure in front of the individual, in the direction of movement, and a low pressure region behind, where the laminar flow of the water is replaced by the turbulent flow. Wave resistance is caused by the body colliding with the waves that are produced by its progression through the water or by movement near the surface, especially up and down movements of body segments. Finally, friction is due to the resistance offered by water immediately upon coming into contact with the body. Therefore, the person's skin, the amount of hair, swimwear and swim speed matters [50].

Therapeutic effects of hydrotherapy:

- To relieve pain and muscle spasm
- To gain relaxation
- To improve proprioception
- To maintain or increase the range of joint movement
- To re-educate paralysed muscles
- To strengthen weak muscles and to develop their power and endurance
- To encourage walking and other functional and recreational activities and reduce re-injury risks
- To improve circulation
- To give the patient encouragement and confidence in carrying out his exercises, thereby improving his morale [43 and 47]

Contra-indications for hydrotherapy:

• Cardiovascular disease	Skin conditions
• Cardiopulmonary disease	Chemical allergies (chlorine)
• Diabetes	Cancer
• Balance disorder	Contagious diseases
• History of cerebrovascular accident, epilepsy	Hepatitis
• Incontinence, urinary tract infection	Urinary incontinence
• Labyrinthitis	Open wounds
• Influenza	Recent surgery
• Fever	Hydrophobia [43 and 47]

Ultrasound

Ultrasound (US) remains one of the most common electrotherapy tools used by sport therapists in their daily clinical practice. It is used in all stages of the healing process and its action is based on the application of acoustic energy to the tissues (Figure 5.8). In other words, these are high frequency sound waves that cannot be perceived by the human ear [51]. Ultrasound travels mainly in longitudinal waves causing compression and rarefaction due to the fluid nature of the soft tissues.

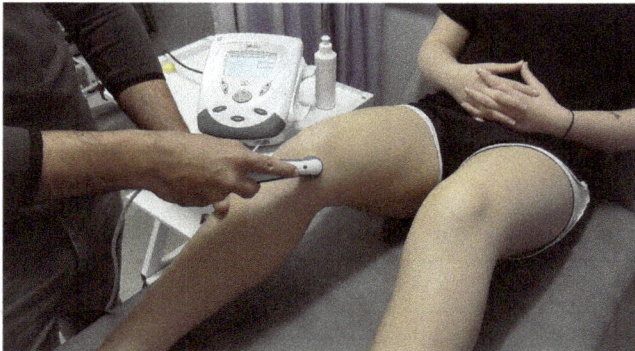

FIGURE 5.8 Ultrasound application.

On the other hand, when ultrasound waves come in contact with the bones, they can also create transverse waves [52]. According to recent systematic reviews, the effectiveness of the ultrasound is based on its proper application and the appropriate parameters [53]. Ultrasound, (Figure 5.8) like any other electrotherapeutic modality, bases its effectiveness on the proper application of its operating parameters which are:

- the frequency of the device
- the type of ultrasound
- the intensity
- the duration of the session
- and the frequency of treatments

The desired ultrasound **frequency** is generated by the inverse or indirect piezoelectric effect and is usually 1MHz or 3MHz. The frequency of 1 MHz shows greater penetration and lower absorbency, while the exact opposite results show the frequency of 3MHz commonly used in daily clinical practice [54].

The **type** of ultrasound can be continuous or intermittent (pulsed). Continuous ultrasound means that all the energy (100%) reaches the tissues, achieving thermal results, while intermittent ultrasound means that part of the energy reaches the tissues in order to produce non-thermal results. In acute injury 1:4 pulse ultrasound is used while in chronic injury it is 1:1.

The **intensity** of the ultrasound ranges between 0.1 and 0.8 W/cm², depending on the type of ultrasound and the desired results. If intermittent ultrasound is used to achieve non-thermal results the intensity is low, and more specifically ranges between 0.1 and 0.3 W/cm². In the subacute stage between 0.2 and 0.5 W/cm² and in the chronic stage between 0.3 and 0.8 W/cm² [55].

Regarding the **duration** of the ultrasound application, the therapist should aim for 1 minute of ultrasound per treatment head area. Therefore, longer time is required if pulsed ultrasound is used and for larger treatment areas. The treatment time that the ultrasound will be applied is given by the equation: Treatment time = 1 x (no. of times treatment head fits onto tissue to treat) x (pulse factor). To determine the pulse factor the therapist needs to add the two components of the ratio together (e.g. – Pulsed at 1:4 adds up to 5, multiply by 5. Pulsed at 1:1, adds up to 2, multiply by 2). The pulse depends on the chronicity of the condition and can be found in the table below (Table 5.3) [55].

With regard to **frequency of treatments**, in acute injuries ultrasound can be applied twice daily, as long as there is at least 6 hours between the applications. In chronic injuries, ultrasound is applied every other day. The total number of sessions depends on the results of the application [56].

The coupling media used in this context include water, various oils, creams and gels. Ideally, the coupling medium should be fluid so as to fill all available spaces, relatively viscous so that it stays in place, have an impedance appropriate to the media it connects, and should allow transmission of US with minimal absorption, attenuation or disturbance. In addition to the reflection that occurs

TABLE 5.3 Suggested ultrasound pulse (Duty Cycle %) according to the chronicity of the condition

Most acute				Most chronic
Pulsed 1:4	Pulsed 1:3	Pulsed 1:2	Pulsed 1:1	Continuous
20%	25%	33%	50%	100%

at a boundary due to differences in impedance, there will also be some refraction if the wave does not strike the boundary surface at 90°, therefore; it is important to keep the ultrasound head at 90°.

Indications for Ultrasound

Ultrasound is indicated for conditions that benefit from the application of deep heat, relief of pain, muscle spasms and joint contractures. The objective of therapeutic ultrasound in the treatment of selected medical conditions associated with the chronic and sub chronic conditions of bursitis/capsulitis, epicondylitis, ligament sprains, tendinitis, scar tissue healing and muscle strain, is to improve healing and reduce pain.

Contra-indications for ultrasound:

• Eyes/gonads – do not use on these areas	Pacemakers
• Pregnancy – avoid the uterus	Altered sensation
• Tumours – can increase tumour growth	Vascular problems
• Growth plates	Active bleeding
• Infections	Metal implant
	Epilepsy

Interferential Current

Interferential current (IFC) therapy is a modality that has been widely used in practice for many years. It is a low frequency electrical stimulation used to give a desired physiological effect and is based on summation of two alternating current signals of slightly different frequency. The resultant current consists of a cyclical modulation of amplitude, based on the difference in frequency between the two signals. When the signals are in phase, they summate to an amplitude sufficient to stimulate, but no stimulation occurs when they are out of phase. The beat frequency of IFC is equal to the difference in the frequencies of the two signals. For example, the beat frequency and, hence, the stimulation rate of a dual channel IFC unit with signals set at 4200 and 4100Hz is 100Hz [57] (Figure 5.9).

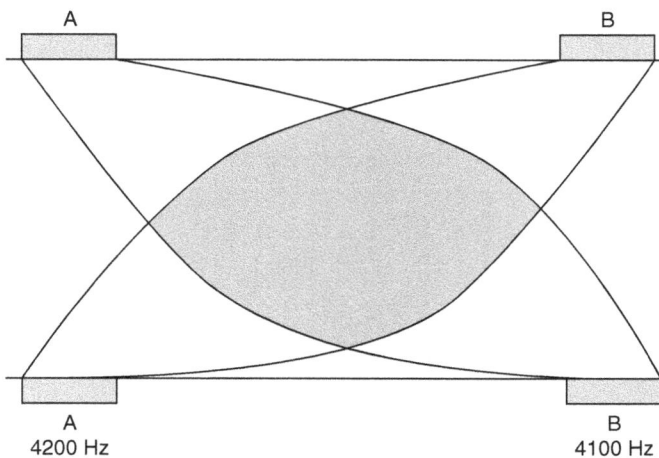

A

B

A
4200 Hz

B
4100 Hz

FIGURE 5.9 The beat frequency generated by current A and current B.

Nerves will accommodate a constant signal and a sweep (gradually changing frequency) is often used to overcome this problem. Sweep occurs between the high and low beat frequency set. The type of sweep used will have a significant effect of the 'stimulation' received by the patient. Most machines offer several sweep patterns, though there is very limited evidence to justify some of these options [55]. There are three main sweep patterns:

- Triangular sweep: gradually changes from the bottom to the top frequencies (equal proportions)
- Rectangular or step sweep: Switches between the top and bottom frequencies rather than a gradual change
- Trapezoid sweep: Combination of the two (Figure 5.10)

The only sweep pattern for which evidence appears to exist is the triangular sweep. The others are perfectly safe to use, but whether they are clinically effective or not remains to be shown.

The basic principle of IFC therapy is to utilise the strong physiological effects of low frequency electrical stimulation of muscle and nerve tissues at sufficient depth without the associated painful and unpleasant side effects of such stimulation. During treatment patient will feel a tingling sensation at the contact area of the electrodes and may also feel the tingling sensation throughout the area being treated. This sensation may continue for a brief period following treatment. Recent research suggests that IFC seems to be very effective on musculoskeletal pain [58] whilst a recent systematic review supports that IFC therapy has the same effects on pain with transcutaneous electrical nerve stimulation (TENS) [59]. Regardless of this evidence, the methodological quality of the studies remains weak and new clinical trials are needed.

Stimulation can be applied using pad electrodes (Figure 5.11) and sponge covers. The sponges should be thoroughly wet to ensure even current distribution. Self-adhesive pad electrodes are also available. Whichever electrode system is employed, electrode positioning should ensure adequate coverage of the area for stimulation. Using larger electrodes will minimise patient discomfort whilst small, closely spaced electrodes increase the risk of superficial tissue irritation and possible damage/skin burn. The bipolar (2 pole) application method is as good as the tetrapolar and there is no physiological difference in treatment outcome [60].

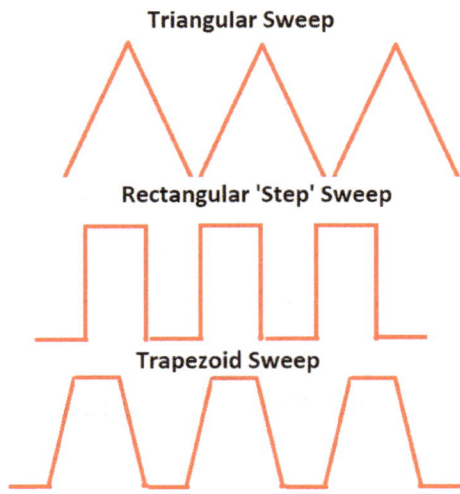

FIGURE 5.10 Interferential current sweep patterns.

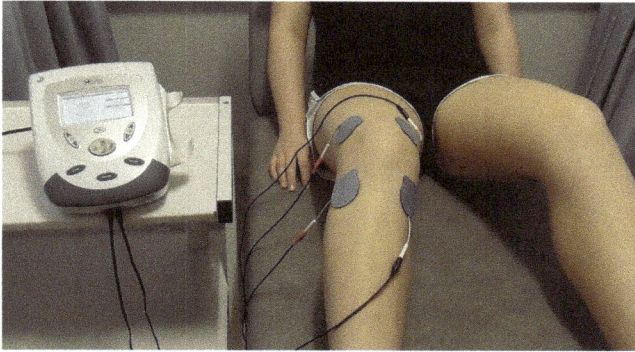

FIGURE 5.11 Interferential treatment with pad electrodes.

There are four main clinical applications for which IFT appears to be used:

*   Pain relief
*   Muscle stimulation
*   Increased local blood flow
*   Reduction of oedema

In addition, claims are made for its role in stimulating healing and repair.

As IFC acts primarily on the excitable (nerve) tissues, the strongest effects are likely to be those which are a direct result of such stimulation (i.e. pain relief and muscle stimulation). The other effects are more likely to be secondary consequences of these.

Pain Relief

IFC is commonly used for pain relief clinically. There are two options in order to achieve pain relief; either with higher frequency (90–130Hz) which stimulates the pain gate mechanism and masks pain symptoms, or, with lower frequency 2–5Hz which activates the bodies localised opioid mechanism, providing a degree of natural pain relief [61–62].

Muscle Stimulation

Stimulation of motor nerves can be achieved through a wide range of frequencies. Low frequency (10Hz) will result in a series of twitches, whilst a higher frequency at 50Hz will result on tetanic contraction. There is limited evidence for the 'strengthening' effect of IFC though Bircan et al. [63] suggest it is possible. On the basis of the current evidence, the contraction brought about by IFC is no 'better' than would be achieved through exercise. The most effective range for Motor Neuron Stimulation is thought to be 10–25Hz.

Increased Local Blood Flow

There is very little (if any) evidence demonstrating a direct effect if IFC on local blood flow changes. Most blood flow measurements are superficial, not deep within the muscle. The most likely option to achieve local blood flow is through the muscle stimulation/contraction. Therefore, the 10–20 or 10–25Hz frequency sweep options appear to be the most likely beneficial option.

Reduction of Oedema

IFC has been claimed to be effective as a treatment to promote the reabsorption of oedema in the tissues. However, there is very limited evidence regarding the physiological mechanisms. Clinical preference is to use IFC for local muscle contraction. Local vascular changes associated with muscle contraction result in increased reabsorption of tissue fluid [55].

Treatment Time

The treatment time varies widely according to the usual clinical parameters of acute/chronic conditions and the type of physiological effect desired. In acute conditions, shorter treatment times of 5–10 minutes may be sufficient to achieve the effect. Longer times may exacerbate the symptoms. Time can be increased if the aim has not been achieved and no untoward side effects have been produced. There is no research evidence to support the continuous progression of a treatment dose in order to increase or maintain its effect. The usual treatment time that is suggested is 10–20 mins, 2–4 per week for a total of 12 weeks.

Contra-indications for interferential current:

- Uncooperative patients
- Fragile or bruised skin
- Under anticoagulation therapy
- History of pulmonary embolism
- Deep vein thrombosis (DVT)

Shock Wave Therapy

A relatively new player in the arsenal of electrophysical therapeutic modalities available for treatment is the extra corporeal shock wave therapy (ECSWT). It was, however, used to break down kidney stones non-invasively in the 1970s. These waves are supersonic in nature. They can be created in our tissue with this device as it creates these supersonic waves via oscillation of the tissue upon contact. It is a form of energy and like any other form of energy when introduced into a human body it will become absorbed differentially depending on the tissue type and density of said tissue. In this sense the waves behave and look quite similar to the sinusoidal wave seen in therapeutic ultrasound. As with all therapeutic modalities it works on the principle of introducing more energy into the target tissue and in so doing so increase the innate metabolic functions of the tissue and thereby optimise and hopefully accelerate tissue repair following injury.

Shockwave therapy is thought to be best used on chronic injuries. It brings the tissue into an acute state much the same as transverse frictions would when applied to superficial thick scar tissue. It is said to also have the ability to: increase local blood flow, increase cellular activity including inflammatory cytokines.

Common clinical application parameter as advised by Watson [55] are as follows.

Treatment Dose Issues

- In addition to the applied energy (mJ/mm2) – in therapy we are using the LOW (up to 0.08mJ/mm2) and possibly the MEDIUM (up to 0.28mJ/mm2) energy levels, the other significant factors are
  - number of shocks and
  - number of treatment session repetitions

Shock Number

- Shock number usually between 1,000 and 1,500, though some authorities suggest up to 2,000
- Some research has tried as few as 100 and also 500
- 500 more effective than 100
- 1,000–1,500 have been used in the clinical trials with the best (most significant) outcomes
- Anecdotally, 1,000–2,000 shocks per session appears to be the most commonly applied range

This modality has robust evidence for its use on tendinopathies, i.e. Achilles, patellar, supraspinatus, biceps (both brachial and femoral) and is most commonly used on plantar fasciitis.

Typically, 3–5 sessions appear to be effective for the majority of patients, spaced such as to let the tissue 'reaction' at least partly subside from the first session before the next treatment is delivered. As with all modalities, a comprehensive past medical history should be taken prior to the application of the selected electrotherapeutic modality the clinician feels best suits the individual's rehabilitation requirements at the time of the therapy session. This is necessary in order to exclude any contra-indications of this and any other modality prior to its application.

Contra-indications for ECSWT:

- Haemophilia
- Malignancies
- Infections (internal or on skin at point of local application)
- Loss of sensation

Instrument-Assisted Soft Tissue Mobilisation (IASTM)

Instrument-assisted soft tissue mobilisation (IASTM) is a new range of tool of specialised soft tissue mobilisation (Figure 5.12). There are several variations of this equipment from different manufacturing companies (myobar, fibroblaster, K-tools, Hawk Grips, Smart tools, Zuka tools, Graston Technique). The technique itself is said to be a modern evolution from traditional Chinese medicine called GuaSha. IASTM is a procedure that is rapidly growing in popularity due to its effectiveness and efficiency while remaining non-invasive, with its own indications and limitations. IASTM is performed with ergonomically designed instruments that detect and treat fascial restrictions,

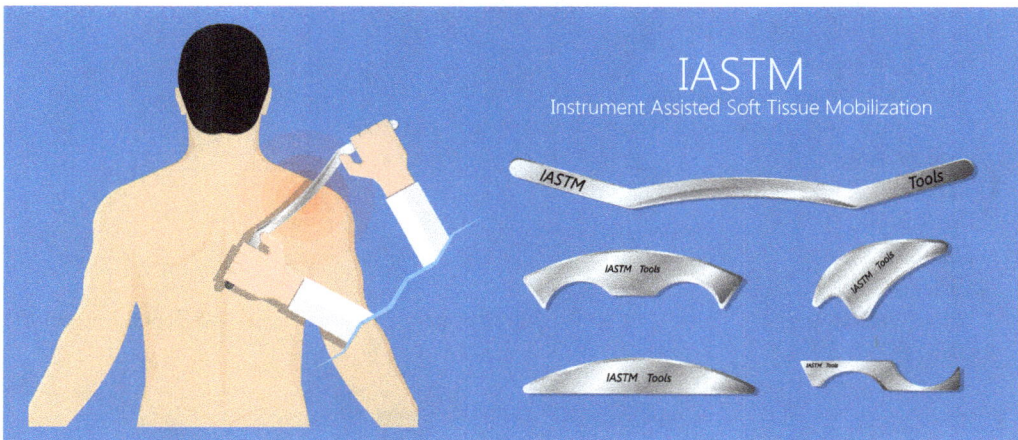

FIGURE 5.12   The instrument-assisted technique.

encourage rapid localisation and effectively treat areas exhibiting soft tissue fibrosis, chronic inflammation or degeneration. The IASTM technique (Figure 5.12) can be issued in tandem with other modalities or exercises.

How Does IASTM Work?

Instruments effectively break down fascial restrictions and scar tissue. The instruments have an ergonomic design which provide the clinician with the ability to locate restrictions and treat the affected area with the appropriate amount of pressure.

The technique causes controlled micro-trauma to the affected soft tissue structure. This micro-trauma causes the stimulation of a local inflammatory response. The IASTM application initiates reabsorption of inappropriate fibrosis, realigns the new fibres and facilitates a cascade of healing activities resulting in remodelling of affected soft tissue structures. The technique can be used after surgery where adhesions within the soft tissue may have been developed due to immobilisation, repeated strain or other mechanisms. IASTM aims to break them down allowing full restoration [64–65]. A recent systematic review provides support for IASTM in improving ROM in uninjured individuals as well as pain and patient-reported function (or both) in injured patients; however, the quality of studies needs to be improved in order to further substantiate and allow for generalisation of these findings [66].

Indications for IASTM

Currently, there is no consensus on the optimal IASTM intervention including type of instrument, stroke technique, treatment parameters (e.g. time, angle, cadence) or applied pressure. Despite the lack of universal agreement on optimal treatment parameters, the existing literature does support the use of IASTM as a treatment when the aim is to:

- Increase range of motion
- Decrease pain during motion
- Treat motor control issues
- Increase muscle recruitment.

Contra-Indications for IASTM

The contra-indications include specific medical conditions, such as but not limited to:

- High pain sensation
- Acute inflammatory conditions
- Congestive heart disease/circulatory disorders
- Osteoporosis
- Cancer
- Pregnancy
- Diabetes
- Varicose veins
- Hypertension, may be considered either precautionary or contraindicative depending on the client [67]

References

1. Nd Do, C. M. (2004). *Handbook of clinical massage: A complete guide for students and practitioners* (2nd ed.) Edinburgh, New York: Churchill Livingstone.
2. Holey, E., & Cook, E. (2003). *Evidence-based therapeutic massage: A practical guide for therapists* (2nd ed.). Edinburgh: Churchill Livingstone.
3. Samples, P. (1987). Does 'sports massage' have a role in sports medicine?. *The Physician and sportsmedicine, 15*(3), 177–183. https://doi.org/10.1080/00913847.1987.11709311
4. Ryan, A. J. (1980). The neglected art of massage. *The physician and sportsmedicine, 8*(12), 25. https://doi.org/10.1080/00913847.1980.11948662
5. Stamford, B. (1985). Massage for athletes. *The Physician and sportsmedicine, 13*(10), 178. https://doi.org/10.1080/00913847.1985.11708915
6. Benjamin, P. J., & Lamp, S. P. (1996). *Understanding sports massage.* Champaign, IL: Human Kinetics.
7. Spina, A. A. (2007). External coxa saltans (snapping hip) treated with active release techniques: a case report. *The Journal of the Canadian Chiropractic Association, 51*(1), 23–29.
8. Yuill, E. A., & Macintyre, I. G. (2010). Posterior tibialis tendonopathy in an adolescent soccer player: a case report. *The Journal of the Canadian Chiropractic Association, 54*(4), 293–300.
9. Simons, D. G., Travell, J. G., Simons, L. S., & Travell, J. G. (1999). *Travell & Simons' myofascial pain and dysfunction: The trigger point manual.* Baltimore, MD: Williams & Wilkins.
10. Batavia, M. (2004). Contraindications for therapeutic massage: do sources agree?. *Journal of bodywork and movement therapies, 8*(1), 48–57.
11. Braverman, D. L., & Schulman, R. A. (1999). Massage techniques in rehabilitation medicine. *Physical medicine and rehabilitation clinics of North America, 10*(3), 631–ix.
12. Park, H., Jeong, T., & Lee, J. (2017). Effects of sling exercise on flexibility, balance ability, body form, and pain in patients with chronic low back pain. *Rehabilitation nursing: the official journal of the Association of Rehabilitation Nurses, 42*(6), E1–E8. https://doi.org/10.1002/rnj.287
13. Saal, J. S. (1998). Flexibility training. In Kibler, W. B., Herring, S. A., & Press, J. M. (eds), *Functional rehabilitation of sports and musculoskeletal injuries.* Gaithersburg, MD: Aspen.
14. Cipriani, D., Abel, B., & Pirrwitz, D. (2003). A comparison of two stretching protocols on hip range of motion: implications for total daily stretch duration. *Journal of strength and conditioning research, 17*(2), 274–278. https://doi.org/10.1519/1533–4287(2003)0172.0.co;2
15. Taylor, D. C., Dalton, J. D. Jr., Seaber, A. V., & Garrett, W. E. Jr. (1990). Viscoelastic properties of muscle-tendon units. The biomechanical effects of stretching. *The American journal of sports medicine, 18*(3), 300–309. https://doi.org/10.1177/036354659001800314
16. Page, P. (2012). Current concepts in muscle stretching for exercise and rehabilitation. *International journal of sports physical therapy, 7*(1), 109–119.
17. Mason, D. (2014). Exercise in rehabilitation. In Porter, S. (ed.), *Tidy's physiotherapy.* London: Elsevier Health Sciences.
18. Page, P., Frank, C. C., Lardner, R., & Human Kinetics. (2014). Assessment and treatment of muscle imbalance: The Janda approach. Champaign, IL: Human Kinetics.
19. Torres, E. M., Kraemer, W. J., Vingren, J. L., Volek, J. S., Hatfield, D. L., Spiering, B. A., Ho, J. Y., Fragala, M. S., Thomas, G. A., Anderson, J. M., Häkkinen, K., & Maresh, C. M. (2008). Effects of stretching on upper-body muscular performance. *Journal of strength and conditioning research, 22*(4), 1279–1285. https://doi.org/10.1519/JSC.0b013e31816eb501
20. Pearce, A. J., Kidgell, D. J., Zois, J., & Carlson, J. S. (2009). Effects of secondary warm up following stretching. *European journal of applied physiology, 105*(2), 175–183. https://doi.org/10.1007/s00421-008-0887-3
21. Barnes, J. F. (1990). *Myofascial release: The search for excellence: A comprehensive evaluatory and treatment approach.* Paoli, PA: J.F. Barnes.
22. McKenney, K., Elder, A. S., Elder, C., & Hutchins, A. (2013). Myofascial release as a treatment for orthopaedic conditions: a systematic review. *Journal of athletic training, 48*(4), 522–527. https://doi.org/10.4085/1062-6050-48.3.17
23. Schleip, R. (January 1, 2003). Fascial plasticity – a new neurobiological explanation: part 1. *Journal of bodywork and movement therapies, 7*(1), 11–19.

24. Klingler, W., Velders, M., Hoppe, K., Pedro, M., & Schleip, R. (2014). Clinical relevance of fascial tissue and dysfunctions. *Current pain and headache reports, 18*(8), 439. https://doi.org/10.1007/s11916-014-0439-y

25. Ajimsha, M. S., Al-Mudahka, N. R., & Al-Madzhar, J. A. (2015). Effectiveness of myofascial release: systematic review of randomized controlled trials. *Journal of bodywork and movement therapies, 19*(1), 102–112. https://doi.org/10.1016/j.jbmt.2014.06.001

26. Laimi, K., Mäkilä, A., Bärlund, E., Katajapuu, N., Oksanen, A., Seikkula, V., Karppinen, J., & Saltychev, M. (2018). Effectiveness of myofascial release in treatment of chronic musculoskeletal pain: a systematic review. *Clinical rehabilitation, 32*(4), 440–450. https://doi.org/10.1177/0269215517732820

27. Sullivan, K. M., Silvey, D. B., Button, D. C., & Behm, D. G. (2013). Roller-massager application to the hamstrings increases sit-and-reach range of motion within five to ten seconds without performance impairments. *International journal of sports physical therapy, 8*(3), 228–236.

28. Jay, K., Sundstrup, E., Søndergaard, S. D., Behm, D., Brandt, M., Særvoll, C. A., Jakobsen, M. D., & Andersen, L. L. (2014). Specific and cross over effects of massage for muscle soreness: randomized controlled trial. *International journal of sports physical therapy, 9*(1), 82–91.

29. Bradbury-Squires, D. J., Noftall, J. C., Sullivan, K. M., Behm, D. G., Power, K. E., & Button, D. C. (2015). Roller-massager application to the quadriceps and knee-joint range of motion and neuromuscular efficiency during a lunge. *Journal of athletic training, 50*(2), 133–140. https://doi.org/10.4085/1062-6050-49.5.03

30. Seffinger, M. A., & Hruby, R. J. (2007). *Evidence-based manual medicine: A problem-oriented approach.* Philadelphia, PA: Saunders/Elsevier.

31. Aboushanab, T. S., & AlSanad, S. (2018). Cupping therapy: an overview from a modern medicine perspective. *Journal of acupuncture and meridian studies, 11*(3), 83–87. https://doi.org/10.1016/j.jams.2018.02.001

32. Liu, W., Piao, S.-A., Meng, X.-W., & Wei, L.-H. (2013). Effects of cupping on blood flow under skin of back in healthy human. *World Journal of Acupuncture – Moxibustion, 23*(3), 50–52.

33. Saha, F. J., Schumann, S., Cramer, H., Hohmann, C., Choi, K. E., Rolke, R., Langhorst, J., Rampp, T., Dobos, G., & Lauche, R. (2017). The effects of cupping massage in patients with chronic neck pain – a randomised controlled trial. *Complementary medicine research, 24*(1), 26–32. https://doi.org/10.1159/000454872

34. Emerich, M., Braeunig, M., Clement, H. W., Lüdtke, R., & Huber, R. (2014). Mode of action of cupping–local metabolism and pain thresholds in neck pain patients and healthy subjects. *Complementary therapies in medicine, 22*(1), 148–158. https://doi.org/10.1016/j.ctim.2013.12.013

35. Khalil, A., AlQaoud, K., & Shaqqour, H. (2013). Investigation of selected immunocytogenetic effects of wet cupping in healthy men. *Spatula Dd – Peer Reviewed Journal on complementary medicine and drug discovery, 3*(2), 51.

36. Guo, Y., Chen, B., Wang, D. Q., Li, M. Y., Lim, C. H., Guo, Y., & Chen, Z. (2017). Cupping regulates local immunomodulation to activate neural-endocrine-immune worknet. *Complementary therapies in clinical practice, 28*, 1–3. https://doi.org/10.1016/j.ctcp.2017.04.005

37. Al-Bedah, A., Aboushanab, T. S., Alqaed, M., Qureshi, N., Suhaibani, I., Ibrahim, G., & Khalil, M. (10 January 2016). Classification of cupping therapy: a tool for modernization and standardization. *Journal of complementary and alternative medical research, 1*(1), 1–10.

38. Edmond, S. L. (1993). *Manipulation and mobilization: Extremity and spinal techniques.* St. Louis, MO: Mosby.

39. A tribute to the life and work of G. D. Maitland 1924–2010 by the International Maitland Teachers Association. (2010). *Manual therapy, 15*(3), 300–301.

40. Levangie, P. K., & Norkin, C. C. (2005). *Joint structure and function: A comprehensive analysis* (4th ed.) Philadelphia, PA: F.A. Davis Co.

41. Kaltenborn, F. M., Evjenth, O., Kaltenborn, T. B., Morgan, D., & Vollowitz, E. (2002). *Manual mobilization of the joints: The Kaltenborn method of joint examination and treatment; Volume I: The extremities.* Oslo: Olaf Norlis Bokhandel.

42. Hengeveld, E., & Banks, K. (2014). *Maitland's peripheral manipulation: Management of neuromusculoskeletal disorders: Volume two.* London: Elsevier Health Sciences.

43. Kamioka, H., Tsutani, K., Okuizumi, H., Mutoh, Y., Ohta, M., Handa, S., Okada, S., Kitayuguchi, J., Kamada, M., Shiozawa, N., & Honda, T. (2010). Effectiveness of aquatic exercise and balneotherapy: a summary of systematic reviews based on randomized controlled trials of water immersion therapies. *Journal of epidemiology, 20*(1), 2–12. https://doi.org/10.2188/jea.je20090030

44. Wilk, K. E., & Joyner, D. M. (2014). *The use of aquatics in orthopedics and sports medicine rehabilitation and physical conditioning.* Thorofare, NJ: Slack.

45. Harrison, R., & Bulstrode, S. (1987). Percentage weight-bearing during partial immersion in the hydrotherapy pool. *Physiotherapy practice, 3*(2), 60–63.

46. Ruoti, R. G., Morris, D. M., & Cole, A. J. (1997). *Aquatic rehabilitation.* Philadelphia, PA: Lippincott.

47. Meeusen, R. (2003). *Aquatherapie.* Mechelen: Kluwer.

48. Edlich, R. F., Towler, M. A., Goitz, R. J., Wilder, R. P., Buschbacher, L. P., Morgan, R. F., & Thacker, J. G. (1987). Bioengineering principles of hydrotherapy. *The Journal of burn care & rehabilitation, 8*(6), 580–584.

49. Dowzer, C. N., Reilly, T., & Cable, N. T. (1998). Effects of deep and shallow water running on spinal shrinkage. *British journal of sports medicine, 32*(1), 44–48. https://doi.org/10.1136/bjsm.32.1.44

50. Torres-Ronda, L., & Del Alcázar, X. S. (2014). The properties of water and their applications for training. *Journal of human kinetics*, 44, 237–248. https://doi.org/10.2478/hukin-2014-0129

51. Erdogan, O., & Esen, E. (2009). Biological aspects and clinical importance of ultrasound therapy in bone healing. *Journal of ultrasound in medicine: official journal of the American Institute of Ultrasound in Medicine, 28*(6), 765–776. https://doi.org/10.7863/jum.2009.28.6.765

52. Haar, G. T., Dyson, M., & Oakley, S. (1 January 1988). Ultrasound in physiotherapy in the United Kingdom: Results of a questionnaire. *Physiotherapy practice, 4*(2), 69–72.

53. Stasinopoulos, D., Cheimonidou, A. Z., & Chatzidamianos, T. (2013) Are there effective ultrasound parameters in the management of lateral elbow tendinopathy? A systematic review of the literature. *Int J phys med rehabil*, 1, 117. doi:10.4172/2329–9096.1000117

54. Draper, D. O., Castel, J. C., & Castel, D. (1995). Rate of temperature increase in human muscle during 1 MHz and 3 MHz continuous ultrasound. *The Journal of orthopaedic and sports physical therapy, 22*(4), 142–150. https://doi.org/10.2519/jospt.1995.22.4.142

55. www.Electrotherapy.org. Accessed 26 August 2020.

56. Watson, T. (2008). *Electrotherapy: Evidence based practice.* London: Elsevier.

57. Moran, F., Leonard, T., Hawthorne, S., Hughes, C. M., McCrum-Gardner, E., Johnson, M. I., Rakel, B. A., Sluka, K. A., & Walsh, D. M. (2011). Hypoalgesia in response to transcutaneous electrical nerve stimulation (TENS) depends on stimulation intensity. *The journal of pain: official journal of the American Pain Society, 12*(8), 929–935. https://doi.org/10.1016/j.jpain.2011.02.352

58. Fuentes, J. P., Armijo Olivo, S., Magee, D. J., & Gross, D. P. (2010). Effectiveness of interferential current therapy in the management of musculoskeletal pain: a systematic review and meta-analysis. *Physical therapy, 90*(9), 1219–1238. https://doi.org/10.2522/ptj.20090335

59. Almeida, C. C., Silva, V., Júnior, G. C., Liebano, R. E., & Durigan, J. (2018). Transcutaneous electrical nerve stimulation and interferential current demonstrate similar effects in relieving acute and chronic pain: a systematic review with meta-analysis. *Brazilian journal of physical therapy, 22*(5), 347–354. https://doi.org/10.1016/j.bjpt.2017.12.005

60. Ozcan, J., Ward, A. R., & Robertson, V. J. (2004). A comparison of true and premodulated interferential currents. Archives of physical medicine and rehabilitation, 85(3), 409–415. https://doi.org/10.1016/s0003-9993(03)00478-7

61. Rocha, C. S., Lanferdini, F. J., Kolberg, C., Silva, M. F., Vaz, M. A., Partata, W. A., & Zaro, M. A. (2012). Interferential therapy effect on mechanical pain threshold and isometric torque after delayed onset muscle soreness induction in human hamstrings. *Journal of sports sciences, 30*(8), 733–742. https://doi.org/10.1080/02640414.2012.672025

62. Atamaz, F. C., Durmaz, B., Baydar, M., Demircioglu, O. Y., Iyiyapici, A., Kuran, B., Oncel, S., & Sendur, O. F. (2012). Comparison of the efficacy of transcutaneous electrical nerve stimulation, interferential currents, and shortwave diathermy in knee osteoarthritis: a double-blind, randomized, controlled, multicenter study. *Archives of physical medicine and rehabilitation, 93*(5), 748–756. https://doi.org/10.1016/j.apmr.2011.11.037

63. Bircan, C., Senocak, O., Peker, O., Kaya, A., Tamci, S. A., Gulbahar, S., & Akalin, E. (2002). Efficacy of two forms of electrical stimulation in increasing quadriceps strength: a randomized controlled trial. *Clinical rehabilitation, 16*(2), 194–199. https://doi.org/10.1191/0269215502cr467oa

64. Fowler, S., Wilson, J. K., & Sevier, T. L. (2000). Innovative approach for the treatment of cumulative trauma disorders. *Work, 15*(1), 9–14.

65. Wilson, J. K., Sevier, T. L., Helfst, R., Honing, E. W., & Thomann, A. (1 November 2000). Comparison of rehabilitation methods in the treatment of patellar tendinitis. *Journal of Sport Rehabilitation, 9*(4), 304–314.

66. Seffrin, C. B., Cattano, N. M., Reed, M. A., & Gardiner-Shires, A. M. (2019). Instrument-assisted soft tissue mobilization: a systematic review and effect-size analysis. *Journal of athletic training, 54*(7), 808–821. https://doi.org/10.4085/1062-6050-481-17

67. Cheatham, S. W., Baker, R., & Kreiswirth, E. (2019). Instrument-assisted soft tissue mobilization: A commentary on clinical practice guidelines for rehabilitation professionals. *International journal of sports physical therapy, 14*(4), 670–682.

6

PRINCIPLES OF EXERCISE AND REHABILITATION

Alex Anzelmo

Exercising correctly with the appropriate equipment, gradation of difficulty/intensity along with appropriate rest, nutrition and hydration protocols are vital in achieving one's goals within exercise (E) and or sport. The importance of physical fitness in humans cannot be overemphasised in relation to its correlation to well-being in man. Several studies demonstrate that there is a correlation between physical fitness and all the positives it delivers i.e. well-being. Higher incidences of cancer occur within individuals that are not physically fit and that have higher levels of adiposity [1–2]. JR Ruiz [3] found that muscular strength, low body fat percentages, and cardiorespiratory fitness adds to the protective effect against cancer mortality.

From this, one must conclude that being 'physically fit' is pivotal to our well-being. So, what is 'fitness'? 'Physical fitness is one's ability to execute daily activities with optimal performance, endurance, and strength with the management of disease, fatigue, stress and reduced sedentary behaviour' [4]. Many authors have chosen to subdivide physical fitness into various constituent components. One such is the USA 'President's Council on Physical Fitness and Sports Definitions for Health, Fitness, and Physical Activity' [5] have subdivided fitness into numerous components.

Common ones are:

- Agility
- Balance
- Cardiovascular endurance (aerobic power)
- Coordination
- Flexibility
- Muscular endurance
- Power/explosive strength (anaerobic power)
- Reaction time
- Strength (maximal, static, dynamic and explosive)
- Speed

Principles of Fitness

There are various regimens that have been proposed over the years by various authors of how to achieve 'physical fitness'. The following is an example of one that encompasses many past authors' expounded regimens that aspire to achieve safe and results driven E programmes. It uses the acronym: **FITT-VP**. The **FITT** principle was first posited in 1975 [5a]. This regimens' components can be implemented into all other regimens. It can be argued that this FITT acronym was taken from sports physiologist pioneers such as Prof. O. Ästrand in the 1960s [6]. **FITT** refers to the type of exercise one performs and how often it is performed. It can be applied to the three main areas of E, 1) Cardiovascular (CV) E for fitness and Weight loss (WL), 2) Strength training and 3) Flexibility. Its constituent letters can be broken down as follows.

The FITT Principle for Cardiovascular Training

F = frequency, i.e. how often one undertakes an E. This is on a per day/week/month basis. It will obviously vary depending on the individuals' aim and goals. An elite athlete will train more than once a day for hours and a retired individual may E once a day for several minutes. This, as with all the subsequent headings, should be tailored to suit the individual's needs.

I = intensity, i.e. the physical stress level at which one E's. This is an important parameter as it is used as a gauge of how hard one is exercising. The simplest way is to take ones hear rate (HR). The simplest way is to use one's fingers and take either the Carotid artery pulse in the neck or the Radial artery pulse in the wrist over a 15-second period. This is then multiplied by 4 to obtain a 'beats per minute' (bpm) value, which is how HR is normally expressed.

T = time, i.e. how long one spends performing said activity. The time one spends performing the activity is important and is activity dependant and depends on what is the desired outcome. There is no point practising sprints over a 100m distance if you want to obtain a good time in the marathon.

T = type, i.e. what form does the E take e.g. Resistance training, running, swimming etc. This, as in the previous sub heading of time, has a dependency on what one wants to achieve. Some cross-benefits can occur from performing a non-sports specific E but in general individuals perform the E that is relevant to them/their sport and their desired goals. An example where cross-benefits can occur irrespective of the sport one practices is performing high-intensity rowing on a rowing ergometer using a Tabata style E regimen [6a]. Performing this high-intensity E regimen will bestow greater aerobic capacity and a greater anaerobic threshold to the individual. This will see the individual being able to tolerate greater stresses in these systems when sprint swimming. Clearly the muscles (M) involved in rowing are recruited in a differential manner than those seen in swimming, i.e. the Ms used in rowing not being switched on in a manner that is most effective for swimming. However, the CV changes obtained from the rowing will see the individual cope with the CV stresses of sprint swimming or any other aerobic/anaerobic E far more readily. The same regimen can be applied to a leg only based Tabata protocol (cycling and running). E specificity to desired goal outcomes is therefore the central premise one must pursue i.e. if one wants to increase M mass, then CV type Es are not going to achieve that goal for you, and resistance training, incorporating the following V & P (volume and progression) adjunct letters to the FITT acronym will lead to the desired results. It is not to say that each desired area is mutually exclusive when it comes to E type. For example, if the desired goal is WL then this is achieved with CV Es that are non-stop, continuous and aerobic in nature, that last for more than 40 mins. S.H Chin [7] found that many authors cited 45–60 mins up to 5 times/week of activity as being optimal for WL. They found greater WL was seen in individuals that combined this E regimen with calorie restriction.

The initials V & P were later added to the 'FITT' acronym and these add a further dimension to the E regimen of:

V = volume, i.e. total amount of exercise performed in a given period e.g. day, week, month etc. This is essentially a parameter of time.

P = progression, i.e. as one's strength, fitness and stamina increase then one needs to change /progress e.g. Increase the weight load in resistance training, increase the time swimming, distance run etc. Performing this stage correctly is particularly crucial for the health care / sport rehabilitator to 'get right' as too much too soon could lead to re-injury. The discussion will now turn to how the FITT-VP acronym can be applied to achieve different areas within 'physical fitness'.

The FITT Principle and Weight Loss

The FITT-VP system is primarily used for WL and this is achieved via CV type E. The acronym can also be used with weighted and stretching E's. These will be dealt with following on from here. The former two can be applied in a CV manner, or in the traditional increase in strength/mass regimen.

WL is such an important area due to globally increasing numbers of obese, that it is easy to find many authors that have investigated appropriate regimens for WL [8–17].

Frequency: This is based on the simple formula of: energy in (Ein, ingested food) – energy out (Eout, ie. activities of daily living and E) should be equal **(Ein – Eout = 0).** Simply put, eating more food that you burn for that day will result in its storage as fat. Eating insufficient food to cover the energy expenditure of that day will result in WL. The importance of maintaining optimal weight for an individual based on height, sex and age are vital for said individual's health and well-being and is exemplified by the overwhelming plethora of research dedicated to this area along with the continual warnings from the WHO and all medical professionals worldwide that ignoring this fundamental balance will inevitably lead to decline in health [8, 10–21].

Intensity: For the exercise intensity to be effective one should consider keeping max HR during the E period at 60–75% of one's own HR max. This HR number is set individually using 220 as the HR max value and then subtracting the individuals age as an approximate barometer for arriving at the 60% value.

Time: Many authors advocate a minimum of 30 mins of non-stop E to observe CV improvements [22]. The average muscle glycogen (MG) stores in the leg Ms is limited [23]. This equates to approximately 20–25 mins at continuous high-intensity levels before a drop off in performance occurs, or a little over 2hrs for steady state E as seen in marathon running [6, 24]. Once this has been depleted (keeping to the brain glycogen requirement shut off limiting minimum), then continuing to E at a steady submaximal rate will result in fat burning as the source of energy needed to drive the M continued energy demands [6, 25–29]. Therefore 30 mins of continual steady state E will see 5–10 mins of fat burning depending on the individual's MG energy storage capacity. As a result, most fitness/aerobic classes are 60 mins in duration to ensure at least a 20 mins element of fat burning E being performed during the class [30–31].

Type: Modern gyms and health clubs now spoil us for choice as to the type of CV E we can undertake all under one roof. Examples are the aerobic/keep fit classes (many variants exist), rowing machines, stair machines, elliptical trainers, upright and recumbent bikes, swimming and treadmills. The type of E used for weight loss will in most instances involve the use of the lower limb Ms. These are the largest M groups found in humans and can withstand the heaviest forces being exerted through them, i.e. body weight.

The FITT Principle and Strength Training

Frequency: A 2–3-day interval should be adopted to allow for the dissipation of delayed onset of M soreness (DOMS) [32–34]. These authors advocated exercising a M group twice a week for maximal benefits. They state 'the current body of evidence indicates that frequencies of training twice a week promote superior hypertrophic outcomes to once a week'. If we take the legs, the chest and arms and then the back as three separate and major M groups that sees resistance training for six out of the seven days in the week. This should then be linked with the appropriate rest intervals between sets for optimal results. Below, a suggested rest interval for Es to be CV in nature is suggested. For strength gains it has been suggested that:

> In the current literature shows that robust gains in M strength can be achieved even with short rest intervals (60 s). However, it seems that longer duration rest intervals (2 min) are required to maximize strength gains in resistance-trained individuals. With regards to untrained individuals, it seems that short to moderate rest intervals (60–120 s) are sufficient for maximizing M strength gains [35].

Intensity: This will vary depending on what is the desired outcome. If mass is the goal, then higher weights (at individuals set/rep max, generally 3–4 sets at 8–10 reps per set) will see the best outcomes. For increased stamina the resultant change needed for this parameter sees a drop in the weight with higher sets and reps being performed. For M strength gains, a number of sets and repetitions are the order of requisite for desired changes to occur. 'The results of this study support resistance E prescription in excess of 4-sets as being the most effective way to train. (i.e. 8–10 sets) for faster and greater strength gains as compared to 1-set training' (a set is when a fixed number of repetitions of the E are performed [36]. It has been stated weights can be used in the FITT-VP system for CV training. This is achieved by reducing the weight to such a level that a high number of sets can be performed (10 or more as per the German volume training principle). By performing these high repetitions with short time recovery periods between sets, it sees the individual elevate their HR into the 60–75% of HR max levels. The timing between sets is achieved by monitoring ones HR and not allowing it to drop below the 60% HR max level. As long as the HR is kept at this percentage of HR max, then this will make this resisted form of FITT E CV in nature.

Time: This will vary depending on the intensity of the E. If the intensity is high, i.e. heavy weights, then a shorter time of workout will result. Sufficient time between E bouts must be given with this high-intensity work out to allow for ATP re-synthesis/ replenishment within the E'd M group [6, 37–39]. These authors cite 60–120 secs as being typically used as a rest/recovery period for optimal mass and strength gains to be achieved and to achieve workable ATP re-synthesis levels. With the lighter weight regimen for a CV type E then the greater than 20–25 mins regimen/E duration cited earlier should be adopted.

Type: Modern gyms and health clubs offer us a multitude of options from free weights on barbells, dumb bells and kettle bells, to weights on pulleys, hydraulic resistance and resistance bands of varying resistances. One can even use one's own body weight to achieve the desired results (pull ups, dips push ups, etc.).

The FITT Principle as Applied to Stretching

As previously stated, the principle of FITT-VP as applied here is dependent on one's goals and level of participation i.e. an elite athlete will stretch daily and several times a day and an amateur enthusiast will typically only stretch whenever they partake of E, i.e. when they go to the gym/home for their workout or a run outside. Some authors have demonstrated that it is detrimental to use any kind of stretching (ballistic, passive or warm up) prior to resistance training [40]. Stretching has also been attributed in contributing to the dissipation of post-E DOMS [41–42].

Stretching can be defined as increasing the range of motion (ROM) around a joint by increasing the elasticity of the joints surrounding soft tissue [43]. This results in increased flexibility and has been associated with reduce injury [43]. It is currently used as part of a warm up and warm down regimen by keen exercisers/athletes. However, it is the main constituent of the E yoga and all its variant forms (ashtanga, bikram, etc.). Here, as in the previously cited resistance and WL areas of training, the application of the FITT-VP principle will vary based on the individual's needs, goals and starting baseline. So, an Olympic gymnast must clearly have great strength combined with flexibility. Such flexibility and overall strength are unnecessary in a marathon runner or an office worker. It does not preclude the latter seeking to achieve the same standards as an Olympic gymnast if that is their goal.

Frequency: It is recommended that it be performed prior to and after E [44–46]. However, there is no consensus on this and there is a paucity of robust empirical evidence to which one can point to for a universally accepted regimen. If one looks at nature as a model, there are many animals (most notably the cat) that always stretch after they have risen from their resting position. We can all agree they are excellent athletes and perhaps we should look to their example as an example.

Intensity: Again here there is much debate as to how this should be performed and can be argued that it will be linked with the other letter T (type) from the FITT-VP acronym. This is dependant, as always, on the individual's needs and goals and the type of stretching involved. The stretching can either be slow, sustained and passive (1) or ballistic/dynamic in nature (2). Again, this is a source of much dispute as to which is of greater benefit. Both ideologies will be outlined. Some authors advocate slow, relaxed and held positions [43, 47]. Other authors advocate reproduction of the activity in a 'ballistic' manner [48]. Other authors advocate against any type of stretching before E [40]. The Cochrane Review in 2017 found 'Stretch does not have clinically important effects on joint mobility' [49]. They based this on individuals with neurological disorders; as such, this finding cannot be extrapolated out to the general public.

In type 1 stretching, an individual moves the limb/body segment into its stretched/elongated position until they feel a strong tension within the M. This should approximate to a 7/10 score [43, 47]. This position can be increased from its initial stop point after a short period of time (generally a few seconds) as the mechanisms involved that create the tension (as a protective mechanism) relax and allow a further elongation of the soft tissue to occur. This type of stretching is also known as PNF (proprioceptive neuromuscular facilitation). The protective mechanisms that exist to avoid damage within the soft tissue are called Golgi tendon organs and M spindles. These organs are also activated and strengthened when M is contracted as seen in strength training and athletic partici-pation [45].

Burgess 2008 [50] found: 'Stretching is commonly used prior to E, as it is thought to reduce the risk of injury. As tendon properties have been shown to be different between genders, it is proposed that stretching will differentially affect the structure'. The study showed that 'Stiffness and Young's modulus' (the mechanical property that measures the stiffness of a material) are correlated and vary between sexes. Young's modulus is a product of measuring the relationship between stress (force per unit area) and strain (proportional deformation) in a material in the linear elasticity regime of a uniaxial deformation) 'were significantly reduced with stretch for both genders. Females showed significantly greater pre- to post stretch decreases in comparison to males'. The study concluded that 'stretching acutely reduces stiffness of the medial gastrocnemius tendon in females and males, with females showing significantly greater change. The observed disparity between genders may be due in part to variations in tendon moment arm and intrinsic differences in tendon composition. These differential changes in tendon mechanical properties have functional, motor control, and injury risk implications'. This study empirically demonstrates positive effects from stretching, but that there is a variation of stretching capabilities between genders. The female being more flexible and achieving greater flexibility end points than their male counterparts when employing the same stretch regimen. The concept of tissue elasticity and plasticity and their relationships to stresses and its relevance to injury will be discussed later.

Time: Great variations in time discrepancies are seen in the literature as to how long should be dedicated to this and anywhere between 5–60 mins is cited [51]. Each individual stretch hold is also variable, with values of 10 seconds to 60 and more being cited [52].

Type: This will follow the same steps outlined in intensity above. As seen above, there is much debate as to which type, if any, is best for which activity and with which phase in the E should a stretch be performed. At the onset of any physical activity it is a good general guideline to warm up the area to be E'd, i.e. gentle jogging or cycling are examples. This increases the tissue temperature slightly enough to increase the tissue plasticity [53].

This warming up phase should be followed by gentler static stretches that elongate the tissue and then a more dynamic type stretch that sees some replication of the desired activity, i.e. there is no point performing push ups to warm up the arms and chest if you are going to engage in a running activity. It is important to make the warmup and stretching phase relevant to the activity that will take place. Therefore, push ups may help in a throwing type activity when they are followed by the previously outlined stretching protocol.

A Description of the Physiological Changes and Adaptations Associated with Different Forms of Exercise

SAID (Specific Adaptation to Imposed Demand)

This idea was first postulated by Henry in 1958 [54]. He proposed the 'Specificity Hypothesis of Motor Learning'. He described how in order to achieve one's desired goals in performance that a six-point series of steps should be:

1. Start at a basic/simple level and then move on to an advanced/complex activity
2. Movement should at first be slow and then progress to fast execution of the slow movement

3. The progression of force used in the movements should start from low force and move to high force
4. Be it duration or distance covered, the activity should start with short duration/ distance and progress to long duration/distance
5. All activities performed should see movements performed bilaterally to unilaterally
6. As skill and strength acquisition increases within an individual, then in order to see safe and incremental improvements in performance, a gradual use the 'Overload Principle' must be applied

Agreement is hard to find within healthcare and exercise professionals regarding SAID. Clearly it will vary from one individual to another but an ideal on how many sets and repetitions to achieve a goal are needed are impossible to find a consensus on within the literature. Swift [55] states that the activity sets and repetitions-based concept can be applied to the three areas of E: resistance, CV and lastly stretching E's. Most E routines and E professionals will advocate 3–4 sets at 6–10 reps per set when using resistance type E's. It can equally be applied to the other two areas. For example, a sprinter type athlete will typically perform repeated sprint bouts of their distance (typically 100m, 200m and 400m) during their training session. Elite swimmers will swim up to 10,000m a day in training. There is not such a distance event in swimming but this excessive regimen gives the swimmer the time to develop perfect stroke, body positioning technique and the stamina needed to perform multiple races at their chosen events as will be seen in the qualifying round stages that all the various athletes will have to go through to bring the large number of competitor numbers down to the fastest, highest and longest jumpers/throwers athletes as seen in major championship events.

In resistance training (RT) the ideology is based on an individual's ability to perform a 6–10 reps of one's 1 repetition max weighted E. There is no statistical basis for stating more than three sets and yet it is commonly performed [56]. They state:

> RT for upper body M hypertrophy (UBMH) typically entails high volumes of sets per M group per training session. Most RT regimens do not discriminate between upper and lower body M groups, while these groups may respond differently to RT set volumes in terms of maximum skeletal M mass gain. Recent studies have examined the effect of different set volumes on the extent of UBMH to formulate optimal RT regimens and to make RT programmes more time-efficient.

The authors concluded that:

> statistically, high set volumes (≥3) are not significantly better than low set volumes (<3) in regard to UBMH in untrained subjects. For trained subjects, the literature is lacking in well-designed studies comparing low and high training volumes, as well as analysing upper and lower body M separately. Therefore, it is not possible to conclude that high volume of sets offers better results than low volume of sets for UBMH, and vice versa'. This is in stark contrast to the previously cited research [36].

Despite this latest information coaches, personal trainers, on-line training guru's, etc., typically advocate higher sets for trained individuals and the 3 sets 10 reps for novice/untrained individuals. It is clear the dissemination of latest best practice is not being taken up by the exercise professionals and better strategies to have this latest information conveyed to grass roots coaching/training needs to evolve. There are various changes that occur within each of the three areas of RT which leads to M hypertrophy, CV Es which sees enhanced and more efficient neurochemical pathways develop and lastly within stretching tissue plasticity and elasticity is altered. When applying the SAID acronym to M hypertrophy, this occurs when the acto-myosin cross bridges within the M contractile unit are ripped apart, as seen in heavy weighted sessions. This leads to repair of said bridges in the new elongated and enlarged positions that resulted from the tearing due to the M tissue material strength being exceeded during the RT [57–62]. In any of the three areas of strength, CV and flexibility training programmes, the goal is to deliver optimum training and recovery in order to lead to an adaptation within the requisite area. This will lead to improved strength and improved performance. Therefore, determining a tailored regimen of optimal training and recovery is of paramount importance to understanding training efficacy. As seen from the research above there is no gold standard in programming for strength gains, and it should always be tailored to suit the individual athletes' requirements and physiology. However, the principle of progressive overload underlies any successful programme. This is not just in RT but also in complexity of movement. This is exemplified in a gymnast's movement. We have all seen the amazing feats a gymnast can perform on their floor routines where they can not only produce various airborne somersaults but also rotate about an axis in the opposite direction and then land on both feet. Clearly, they do not start by practising this move as they will physically be unprepared to perform this and will not have the ability to control their body to move in these myriads of movements. This end product is the result of daily practice sessions lasting up to 8 hrs a day, 6 days a week across several years adding incremental movements that go to complete the end product we see in the Olympic Games.

Progressive overload is defined as progressively placing greater than normal demands on the exercising M, typically through manipulation of training frequency, volume and intensity [63]. In order to continue to adapt, the body must be subjected to greater stress than before, 'shocking' the neuromuscular system into response and adaptation. While the level of this response and adaptation to any programme is specifically individualised. This premise has been documented in the literature as long ago as 1952 [64]. It stated a consistent, systemic response to all types of stress (weighted/resistance type Es) are a key ingredient to all individuals that wish to either partake in sports or exercise for health benefits or competitive reasons. The strengthening of the appropriate M groups will see an improvement in skill and ultimately performance. An example is a gymnast or dancer needs considerable core and leg strength in order to elevate a leg out from the body up into a vertical position and hold it there. This must be achieved whilst maintaining a perfectly straight leg in a smooth and controlled motion. This can only be achieved if the relevant M's in the supporting leg are strong enough to hold the individual perfectly still and the elevated leg is reciprocally strengthened and flexible enough to position itself in the elevated end point. This, and the majority of movements, will not be possible unless the joint is centrally stabilised, i.e. core strength. Many regimens abound that can be considered in order to achieve M strength/hypertrophy gains. The following two are the most widely used.

Rehabilitation Principles and Stages of Training

DeLorme Technique (DL)

This is a method of E with weights for the purpose of strengthening M in which sets of repetitions are repeated with rests between sets [65]. The technique involves isotonic E and determination of the maximum level of resistance [66].

DAPRE

The Daily Adjustable Progressive Resistive Exercise (**DAPRE**) technique was developed clinically, in an effort, to provide an objective means of increasing resistance concurrently with strength increases during knee rehabilitation subsequent to injury/surgery [67]. This technique is based on the concept of systematic progression such as a periodized strength training regimen where training variables (rest, overall training volume, sets per workout, repetitions per set, and intensity of training) are manipulated over a period of time in order to optimize adaptations to training [68]. As with all the aforementioned acronyms, this one can also be adjusted to an individual's needs and can be applied across the three areas of strength, flexibility and CV E.

The DL technique was developed in 1945 by a US army physician that saw many soldiers returning from WWII with varying levels of orthopaedic injuries. DL himself suffered from a childhood illness that left him weakened (rheumatic fever). He adopted a weighted exercise regimen in order to overcome his post illness weakness. He decided that the best way to help the injured soldiers was to have them engage in the same E protocol that had helped him as a child. His protocol consisted of multiple sets of resistance E's in which patients lifted their 10-repetition maximum (i.e. the maximum weighted movement an individual can perform in 10-repetitions). DL later refined his system in 1948 to include 3 progressively heavier sets of 10 repetitions. He referred to the programme as 'Progressive Resistance Exercise'. The results were so successful that his regimen was adopted as the standard form of treatment used in both the military and public setting when attempting to rehabilitate an individual post orthopaedic trauma.

As with many progressions seen in science, medicine and technology, all advancement can point to a common origin. Taking DL as the common origin point of resistance exercise prescriptions to enhance injury recovery and sporting performance, the DAPRE is once such advancement that was built upon the foundation that is the DL technique.

Physiological and Anatomical Limitations of Physical Activity and Exercise

Injury

How does exercising, stretching, resting and hydrating appropriately post physical endeavour along with appropriate body weight based on an individual's height age and sex have a connection with injury? To understand this, it is necessary to view the body and all its constituent parts (bones, ligaments, tendons, M, skin, etc.) as a material. This material can be damaged if its structural integrity is exceeded. The constituent components that make up a human body all have differing structural make ups, strengths and abilities to absorb and withstand forces that are routinely placed upon them. How they cope with these forces will determine how well the body is able to perform. Within man they vary considerably. This variation is not just due to age, where age sees an overall decrement in these structures abilities to perform but also in healthy young individuals it can vary due to the tissue type's structural capabilities to absorb and withstand forces applied through it. We can all appreciate that even if all 20-year olds were of optimal weight and trained exactly the same, the vast majority of them would not be able to run a sub-9.5 seconds 100m race. Genetics will play a major determinant of body form and the sporting ability that body will have.

Therefore, these body constituent parts that are subject to forces will behave differentially to an applied force depending on how they are configured. For an understanding of this we must move from anatomy and physiology, to the area of physics, namely, mechanical physics. How materials (in the human example a material is a tendon, ligament, M, etc.) absorb and dissipate a force will depend on its ability to change relative to said force. This ability is known as the 'Plasticity of materials'. Using example from physics that applies to all materials. Man is made up of materials of different densities, tensile strengths and plasticity/elasticity. This is an important concept for the healthcare/rehabilitator to take on board. Exceeding the limits of a material will result in its failure, i.e. pulling hard enough on a T-shirt will cause it to tear. This is because the shirts' material tensile strength has been exceeded. Applying this principle to bones, M, tendons and ligaments will see the same catastrophic event occur. The integrity threshold of a material however can vary with temperature, i.e. increasing the temperature of the material will also increase the integrity threshold. Hence warm ups are a good idea before engaging in sporting activity form an injury reduction perspective [53].

Even if individuals and athletes follow the above suggested protocols, it is not a recipe for success. Let us take high jumping as an example of how anthropometric dimensions of an individual (anatomical limitations) can dictate their success in a given sport. If we take elite level high jumpers, they are all typically ectomorphs. In a 2015 study it was found the average height of those able to jump over 2.31m was 1.95m in height. We never see a 1.6m endomorph jump over 2.31m. This is due to a combination of biomechanical considerations such as lever length and power generation, i.e. long, powerful legs.

Fitness Testing in Clinical and Field-based Setting

Fitness Testing

Now that the areas of training types have been explored, the discussion must now turn to how does one measure whether the aforementioned E regimens have conveyed any benefits to the individuals receiving said training. As per the training models there are many tests and measures available and will be cited later.

What Is the Purpose of Fitness Testing?

- To identify the strengths and/or weaknesses in a performance. This in turn informs us of the success of a training regimen
- To monitor improvement
- To have a baseline level of fitness
- To gleam deficiencies in order to identify training requirements
- To compare individuals' values against that of the group/national averages
- To motivate individual to better initial values and to set goals
- To provide a variety in the individuals/group training regimen

Therefore, from the above list one must decide what particular aspect of the improvements gained from the E regimen one wants to measure. For example in strength E regimens the easiest way is to see if the one rep max in a particular E (bench press, squat, etc.) has been improved, i.e. day one of a six-week strengthening programme saw individual 'A' bench press 100 kg for their one rep max. Following the six-week programme, 120 kg was achieved, seeing a 20% improvement. Not all testing programmes are as easy as this to employ and require more complex equipment and or staging. For example, CV improvement can be as simple as measuring the time taken to run 'X' metres. The re-test can be what is the time for the same distance following a six-week training programme. The newly recorded and hopefully faster time will give us an improvement in the time the individual is capable of achieving but will not give us an understanding of any CV changes that may have occurred internally to achieve this improved time. For this measure exhaled gas analysis during E will tell us how efficient the individual has become by the percentage of gases exhaled relative to those prior to the training programme. Blood lactate levels or other metabolites may also be used to enable us to demonstrate increased fitness.

Bleep tests, standing jump height/distance tests, one rep max, blood lactate levels, expired air analysis, body fat loss, M mass increase, etc. may all have improved under a well-designed E programme that wants to improve a specific area within the elite athlete/keen exerciser. This is all well and good if one sets those specific goals at the onset of the training programme, but how do these markers then translate into an analysis of improved performance from a play perspective? In the instance of a running, jumping, throwing, swimming, cycling, weightlifting individual this can be as easy as improved times, heights, distances and weights being achieved from previous base lines, but what of team performance? How is this measured? It can be that a football team that has undergone an extensive programme of strengthening, flexibility, CV, agility, proprioception, etc. training will have shown an improvement by scoring more goals, having more possession of the ball, winning more games, etc. There are many ways in which to measure the direct (blood analysis etc.) and indirect (% of ball possession during a game) benefits of improved performance testing following an E programme intervention, one just has to decide which test will meet your desired outcome measures that the implemented programme can achieve.

Return to Play Tests

After having undertaken the arduous and often long journey of rehabilitation from injury (a surgically repaired anterior cruciate ligament will take an average nine-month period from surgery to return to play), the individual will undertake a series of fitness tests that can be contemporaneously used as a return to play test. If the individual can successfully perform said tests without pain and disability, then return to play can be considered following a re-introduction of the player into training regimens where game situation type play occurs (i.e. scrimmaging).

Commonly Used Tests Are:

- Agility – Illinois agility test
- Balance – Stork stand test
- CV endurance (aerobic power) – Multistage fitness test
- Coordination – Wall toss test
- Flexibility – Sit and reach test
- Muscular endurance – Sit-up bleep test
- Power/explosive strength (anaerobic power) – Vertical jump test/standing long jump test
- Reaction time – Ruler drop test
- Maximal strength – One rep max test
- Speed – 30-metre sprint test (acceleration must be eliminated and so a running start of 20 metres is recommended). Record the time between metres 20 and 50 metres

Anaerobic endurance tests:

- RAST (Running-based anaerobic sprint test)
- Cunningham and Faulkner test

Body composition tests:

- Skin fold callipers
- Bioelectrical impedance analysis

Training Techniques

Plyometric Training

Using the protocols outlined in the FITT-VP section, one can apply said protocols to specific training interventions outside those cited therein [e.g. flexibility (stretching)]. An example is with 'plyometric training'. This term was coined in 1920. A US Olympic long-distance runner that observed the superior performances the Russian athletes were having by using this jumping method of warm ups compared to the static stretching pre event methods other athletes were using. In its simplest form it involves jumping. The athlete experiences a force on landing in which the hip, knee and ankle extensor Ms undergo a powerful eccentric contraction (EC). The Ms in and around these joints have to respond explosively (eccentrically), the EC then rapidly becomes an isometric one (when the downward movement stops) and then the concentric contraction (CC) takes place on the upward phase of movement, This must all occur in a minimum amount of time for it to be effective [69].

In the EC phase, the Ms of the legs are involuntarily lengthened, whilst in the CC phase, the M are shortened after being contracted in the eccentric landing phase. Most of the stretching and shortening takes place in the tendons that attach to the M involved rather than in the Ms. They act as a spring whereby the length changes momentarily store the energy to then quickly release it in the concentric phase. Much the same as is seen when you stretch an elastic band and release it to see it propel quickly forward. To perform this type of E the term 'depth jump' was coined. It sees the athlete stands on a raised platform (usually between the heights of 50–80 cm). Due to the rapid change in M activation time seen in this movement and the fact that landing and taking off occurs from one foot, a greater level of proprioception is imbued to the individual by performing this activity. The activity is very simple and sees the athlete simply step out and drop down in a vertical pathway from the raised platform to land on the floor.

Core Stability

Not only is a greater explosive jumping and sprinting ability conveyed to the individual performing this activity but a greater bone mineral density and lower injury occurrence in lower limbs was seen with individuals that practice this regimen [70, 71]. The ability to perform the plyometric E and indeed many others will not be possible if the individual does not have a 'stable core'. Having a strong and stable core has been attributed to improved physical performance [72]. The core is the central region of the body about which all movements must occur. Many of us can relate to having a painful back and being unable to walk due to said pain. The Ms of the core are commonly cited as: the pelvic floor, transversus abdominis, multifidus, internal and external obliques, rectus abdominis, erector spinae (sacrospinalis) the longissimus thoracis and the diaphragm. The secondary core M's are the latissimus dorsi, gluteus maximus and trapezius. It has been stated that the diaphragm, can significantly affect the posture and movement of the individual by influencing the core. This is seen in the extreme ranges of inspiration and expiration [73]. Performing these Es with high repetition rates and sets will see an improvement in the parameters of strength, power, M endurance, speed, agility, quickness and proprioception [74].

Proprioception

Proprioception/kinaesthesia is one's own innate awareness of body position and movement in space [75]. This movement awareness occurs via a network of specialised nerve endings called proprioceptors that are mechanoreceptors found in all Ms and joints of the body. Our central nervous system takes in and processes information from these proprioceptors and other sensory systems such as those seen in the inner ear (vestibular), skin and the eyes. It then outputs an appropriate response relative to the inputs received. This is achieved in a matter of microseconds as is seen in reflexive hand movement away from a noxious stimulus (i.e. pain)

Energy Systems – Aerobic and Anaerobic

Homeostatic MG refreshment post-E is dictated via the type of foods ingested, when and how much are eaten, along with the individual's hydration levels the length of recovery and how much of the energy stores have been depleted in the previous E bout [76–80]. The approximate 2-hr. replenishment/replacement cycle of MG post food ingestion (in particular CHO) was found by numerous authors [81–86]. The quantity of CHO consumed post-E is an important factor in the replenishment of skeletal MG stores. If insufficient CHO is ingested, then MG stores can take 8 to 10 days to return to normal [85]. If the individual is dehydrated, then there will be a lower blood plasma volume. This reduced volume has been found to be significant regarding MG re-synthesis, i.e. there will be lower levels of glycogen (G) replenishment [76].

It has also been found that the addition of electrolytes such as Na^+, K^+ and Cl^- have been found to facilitate greater restoration of fluid retention than water alone does [87]. An optimal hydration level is important post-E, particularly if substantial water and electrolytes have been lost during E [88]. The amount of CHO needed per individual is clearly dependent on anthropometric considerations, i.e. a 100kg-man will need more than a 50kg-female. Numerous studies have found that 1.2 to 1.5 gm CHO per kg body weight/hr was sufficient for MG replenishment. The average skeletal M store 400 mmol·gm-1 wet weight of G [89]. With the proviso that an initial dose of 50 to 75 gm of CHO is taken on immediately following E cessation homeostasis is achieved quicker than if this is delayed [90–93]. If CHO consumption concentrations are below the individual's optimal levels, a combination of CHO and fat in a 2–3:1 ratio respectively can be used as a guide for MG replenishment [91, 94, 95]. A complex CHO diet yielded greater MG storage than simple sugars 24 hrs after E [84]. If one uses blood glucose and insulin levels as a barometer then this certainly holds true. This is because elevated insulin and blood glucose levels are not necessarily associated with the rate of G replenishment, as blood measures will vary in the demands for E'd and non-E'd M [96, 97]. Non-insulin-dependent MG transport increases via E, thus reducing over time post-E regardless of G repletion levels [98]. Even with elevated plasma glucose and insulin levels the rate of G storage slows over time post-E. This fact supports taking on CHO as soon after E as possible to accelerate this [80]. Many athletes take on CHO (in liquid form) during E. This has been shown not to facilitate greater post-E synthesis rates of MG. What taking on CHO during E has been shown to do is it acts as an overall G sparing enabler during E [79]. The G sparring that occurs when one takes on CHO during E is due to the use of the available fat or blood glucose as the body's fuel source for energy production [82]. A combination of fat and CHO has been shown to be optimal for both G sparing and the rate of G synthesis. One study found that ingestion of a 25% glucose polymer drink 2 hrs post-E reduced G synthesis rates down to a 30% as compared to those that consumed the drink immediately post-E [80].

Glycogen is needed to produce ATP, fatigue results when MG has been depleted. This fatigue onset is dependent on the E intensity i.e. the greater the intensity the quicker the G depletion and the quicker the fatigue occurs. As previously stated, taking on board liquid CHO during E (as seen with marathon runners) can increase the time to exhaustion by sparing MG by maintaining blood glucose levels via its during activity ingestion.

It was previously stated that the timing of post-E CHO feeding is critical. This is to take advantage of the increased blood flow seen during E. This increase, however, reduces markedly upon E cessation. During this time the Ms take in greater amounts of glucose which is converted into G within the first hour. The intake levels return to pre-E levels after approximately 2 hrs. That is why taking on board CHO within the 2 hrs post-E is advocated to optimise M re-synthesis of G. Large quantities of simple CHO eaten during this 2-hr window will see faster re-synthesis times than CHO taken outside the 2-hr post-E window. Many authors suggest ingestion of complex CHO 24 hrs after the E bout, as this seems to help keep insulin levels elevated for longer, aiding in the movement of blood glucose into the M for re-synthesis of MG. Combining the consumption of protein with CHO has also been shown to accelerate MG re-synthesis. This is due to the protein reducing the overall glycaemic load of the food. This has the effect of stabilising the insulin spike which naturally occurs after the initial 24 hrs in the long-term G re-synthesis process.

The role that insulin and blood glucose levels play in the re-synthesis of MG is complex. These levels remain consistent throughout the body's bloodstream even when working M's are using both at high intensity or whilst non-exercising M's shut down their utilisation of blood glucose during E [38].

During sporting activity or E, MG is the primary source for energy [99]. The evidence shows that the duration of E is closely related to the amount of G stored in the M [104]. Decreased performance and fatigue are associated with depleted MG levels during endurance events, even when other energy sources are available [101]. Skeletal Ms rely on localised stores of G and whole-body glucose during prolonged/endurance E [102].

The creation of adenosine triphosphate (ATP) is triggered and controlled via the local MG stores. Differing M have differing ability to store MG [103]. Once an exercising M has depleted its stores of MG, it will be replenished via the liver stores or via the consumption and eventual breakdown of food. The latter takes more time and if this is the method of resupply then the E time will be limited whilst awaiting new MG replenishment to occur from the ingested food breakdown. This process can take up to 2 hrs [88, 94, 104]. It must be noted that glycogenolytic capacity of all M (including cardiac) and its actomyosin ATPase activity are regulated in parallel with each other [104].

References

1. Estévez-López, F., Martinez-Tellez, B., & Ruiz, J. R. (2017). Physical fitness and cancer. *The Lancet oncology, 18*(11), e631. https://doi.org/10.1016/S1470-2045(17)30728-3
2. Farrell, S. W., & Willis, B. L. (2012). Cardiorespiratory fitness, adiposity, and serum 25-dihydroxyvitamin D levels in women: the Cooper Center Longitudinal Study. *Journal of women's health (2002), 21*(1), 80–86. https://doi.org/10.1089/jwh.2010.2684

3. Ruiz, J. R., Sui, X., Lobelo, F., Morrow, J. R., Jr., Jackson, A. W., Sjöström, M., & Blair, S. N. (2008). Association between muscular strength and mortality in men: prospective cohort study. *BMJ, 337*(7661), a439. https://doi.org/10.1136/bmj.a439

4. Campbell, N., De Jesus, S., & Prapavessis, H. (2013). Physical fitness. In Gellman M.D., & Turner J.R. (eds), *Encyclopedia of behavioral medicine*. New York: Springer.

5. Corbin, C. B., Pangrazi, R. P., & Franks, B. D. (2002). *President's council on physical fitness and sports definitions for health, fitness, and physical activity.* Washington DC.

5a. Karl, G. & Pescatello, L. S. (1975). *The American College of Sports Medicine (ACSM) guidelines for exercise testing and prescription.* Philadelphia, PA: Wolters Kluwer, Lippincott Williams & Wilkins.

6. Ästrand, P.O., Rodahl, K., Dahl, H. A., & Strømme, B. (1970). *Textbook of work physiology* (1st ed.). New York: McGraw-Hill.

6a. Tabata, I., Nishimura, K., Kouzaki, M., Hirai, Y., Ogita, F., Miyachi, M., & Yamamoto, K. (1996). Effects of moderate-intensity endurance and high-intensity intermittent training on anaerobic capacity and VO2max. *Medicine and science in sports and exercise, 28*(10), 1327–1330. https://doi.org/10.1097/00005768-199610000-00018

7. Chin, S. H., Kahathuduwa, C. N., & Binks, M. (2016). Physical activity and obesity: what we know and what we need to know. *Obesity reviews: an official journal of the International Association for the Study of Obesity, 17*(12), 1226–1244. https://doi.org/10.1111/obr.12460

8. Jensen, M. D., Ryan, D. H., Apovian, C. M., Ard, J. D., Comuzzie, A. G., Donato, K. A., Hu, F. B., Hubbard, V. S., Jakicic, J. M., Kushner, R. F., Loria, C. M., Millen, B. E., Nonas, C. A., Pi-Sunyer, F. X., Stevens, J., Stevens, V. J., Wadden, T. A., Wolfe, B. M., Yanovski, S. Z., & Jordan, H. S. (2014). 2013 AHA/ACC/TOS guideline for the management of overweight and obesity in adults: a report of the American College of Cardiology/American Heart Association Task Force on Practice Guidelines and The Obesity Society. *Circulation, 129*(25 Suppl 2), S102–S138. https://doi.org/10.1161/01.cir.0000437739.71477.ee

9. Spiegelman, B. M., & Flier, J. S. (2001). Obesity and the regulation of energy balance. *Cell, 104*(4), 531–543. https://doi.org/10.1016/s0092-8674(01)00240-9

10. Franz, M. J., VanWormer, J. J., Crain, A. L., Boucher, J. L., Histon, T., Caplan, W., Bowman, J. D., & Pronk, N. P. (2007). Weight-loss outcomes: a systematic review and meta-analysis of weight-loss clinical trials with a minimum 1-year follow-up. *Journal of the American Dietetic Association, 107*(10), 1755–1767. https://doi.org/10.1016/j.jada.2007.07.017

11. Wu, T., Gao, X., Chen, M., & van Dam, R. M. (2009). Long-term effectiveness of diet-plus-exercise interventions vs. diet-only interventions for weight loss: a meta-analysis. *Obesity reviews: an official journal of the International Association for the Study of Obesity, 10*(3), 313–323. https://doi.org/10.1111/j.1467-789X.2008.00547.x

12. Goodpaster, B. H., Delany, J. P., Otto, A. D., Kuller, L., Vockley, J., South-Paul, J. E., Thomas, S. B., Brown, J., McTigue, K., Hames, K. C., Lang, W., & Jakicic, J. M. (2010). Effects of diet and physical activity interventions on weight loss and cardiometabolic risk factors in severely obese adults: a randomized trial. *JAMA, 304*(16), 1795–1802. https://doi.org/10.1001/jama.2010.1505

13. Foster-Schubert, K. E., Alfano, C. M., Duggan, C. R., Xiao, L., Campbell, K. L., Kong, A., Bain, C. E., Wang, C.Y., Blackburn, G. L., & McTiernan, A. (2012). Effect of diet and exercise, alone or combined, on weight and body composition in overweight-to-obese postmenopausal women. *Obesity, 20*(8), 1628–1638. https://doi.org/10.1038/oby.2011.76

14. Curioni, C. C., & Lourenço, P. M. (2005). Long-term weight loss after diet and exercise: a systematic review. *International journal of obesity, 29*(10), 1168–1174. https://doi.org/10.1038/sj.ijo.0803015

15. Villareal, D. T., Chode, S., Parimi, N., Sinacore, D. R., Hilton, T., Armamento-Villareal, R., Napoli, N., Qualls, C., & Shah, K. (2011). Weight loss, exercise, or both and physical function in obese older adults. *The New England journal of medicine, 364*(13), 1218–1229. https://doi.org/10.1056/NEJMoa1008234

16. Donnelly, J. E., Jacobsen, D. J., Heelan, K. S., Seip, R., & Smith, S. (2000). The effects of 18 months of intermittent vs. continuous exercise on aerobic capacity, body weight and composition, and metabolic fitness in previously sedentary, moderately obese females. *Int J obes relat metab disord*, 24, 566–572.

17. Thorogood, A., Mottillo, S., Shimony, A., Filion, K. B., Joseph, L., Genest, J., Pilote, L., Poirier, P., Schiffrin, E. L., & Eisenberg, M. J. (2011). Isolated aerobic exercise and weight loss: a systematic review and

meta-analysis of randomized controlled trials. *The American journal of medicine, 124*(8), 747–755. https://doi.org/10.1016/j.amjmed.2011.02.037

18. Burke, L. M., Cox, G. R., Culmmings, N. K., & Desbrow, B. (2001). Guidelines for daily carbohydrate intake: do athletes achieve them? *Sports medicine, 31*(4), 267–299. https://doi.org/10.2165/00007256-200131040-00003

19. Spiegelman, B. M., & Flier, J. S. (2001). Obesity and the regulation of energy balance. *Cell, 104*(4), 531–543. https://doi.org/10.1016/s0092-8674(01)00240-9

20. Simpson, S. A., Shaw, C., & McNamara, R. (2011). What is the most effective way to maintain weight loss in adults?. *BMJ, 343*, d8042. https://doi.org/10.1136/bmj.d8042

21. Dhurandhar, N. V., Schoeller, D., Brown, A. W., Heymsfield, S. B., Thomas, D., Sørensen, T. I., Speakman, J. R., Jeansonne, M., Allison, D. B., & Energy Balance Measurement Working Group (2015). Energy balance measurement: when something is not better than nothing. *International journal of obesity (2005), 39*(7), 1109–1113. https://doi.org/10.1038/ijo.2014.199

22. Swift, D. L., Johannsen, N. M., Tudor-Locke, C., Earnest, C. P., Johnson, W. D., Blair, S. N., Sénéchal, M., & Church, T. S. (2012). Exercise training and habitual physical activity: a randomized controlled trial. *American journal of preventive medicine, 43*(6), 629–635. https://doi.org/10.1016/j.amepre.2012.08.024

23. Hearris, M. A., Hammond, K. M., Fell, J. M., & Morton, J. P. (2018). Regulation of muscle glycogen metabolism during exercise: implications for endurance performance and training adaptations. *Nutrients, 10*(3), 298. https://doi.org/10.3390/nu10030298

24. Murray, B., & Rosenbloom, C. (2018). Fundamentals of glycogen metabolism for coaches and athletes. *Nutrition reviews, 76*(4), 243–259. https://doi.org/10.1093/nutrit/nuy001

25. Elia, M., Fuller, N. J., & Murgatroyd, P. R. (1992). Measurement of bicarbonate turnover in humans: applicability to estimation of energy expenditure. *The American journal of physiology, 263*(4 Pt 1), E676–E687. https://doi.org/10.1152/ajpendo.1992.263.4.E676

26. Henry, C. J. (2005). Basal metabolic rate studies in humans: measurement and development of new equations. *Public health nutrition, 8*(7A), 1133–1152. https://doi.org/10.1079/phn2005801

27. Boutche, r S. H. (2011). High-intensity intermittent exercise and fat loss. *Journal of obesity, 2011*, 868305. https://doi.org/10.1155/2011/868305

28. Secher, N. H., Seifert, T., & Van Lieshout, J. J. (2008). Cerebral blood flow and metabolism during exercise: implications for fatigue. *Journal of applied physiology, 104*(1), 306–314. https://doi.org/10.1152/japplphysiol.00853.2007

29. Ogoh, S., Dalsgaard, M. K., Yoshiga, C. C., Dawson, E. A., Keller, D. M., Raven, P. B., & Secher, N. H. (2005). Dynamic cerebral autoregulation during exhaustive exercise in humans. *American journal of physiology. Heart and circulatory physiology, 288*(3), H1461–H1467. https://doi.org/10.1152/ajpheart.00948.2004

30. Moghetti, P., Bacchi, E., Brangani, C., Donà, S., & Negri, C. (2016). Metabolic effects of exercise. *Frontiers of hormone research, 47*, 44–57. https://doi.org/10.1159/000445156

31. Watt, M. J., & Cheng, Y. (2017). Triglyceride metabolism in exercising muscle. *Biochimica et biophysica acta. Molecular and cell biology of lipids, 1862*(10 Pt B), 1250–1259. https://doi.org/10.1016/j.bbalip.2017.06.015

32. Hansen, A. K., Fischer, C. P., Plomgaard, P., Andersen, J. L., Saltin, B., & Pedersen, B. K. (2005). Skeletal muscle adaptation: training twice every second day vs. training once daily. *Journal of applied physiology, 98*(1), 93–99. https://doi.org/10.1152/japplphysiol.00163.2004

33. Cheung, K., Hume, P., & Maxwell, L. (2003). Delayed onset muscle soreness: treatment strategies and performance factors. *Sports medicine, 33*(2), 145–164. https://doi.org/10.2165/00007256-200333020-00005

34. Schoenfeld, B. J., Ogborn, D., & Krieger, J. W. (2016). Effects of resistance training frequency on measures of muscle hypertrophy: a systematic review and meta-analysis. *Sports medicine, 46*(11), 1689–1697. https://doi.org/10.1007/s40279-016-0543-8

35. Grgic, J., Schoenfeld, B. J., Skrepnik, M., Davies, T. B., & Mikulic, P. (2018). Effects of rest interval duration in resistance training on measures of muscular Strength: a systematic review. *Sports medicine, 48*(1), 137–151. https://doi.org/10.1007/s40279-017-0788-x

36. Marshall, P. W., McEwen, M., & Robbins, D. W. (2011). Strength and neuromuscular adaptation following one, four, and eight sets of high intensity resistance exercise in trained males. *European journal of applied physiology, 111*(12), 3007–3016. https://doi.org/10.1007/s00421-011-1944-x

37. Hargreaves, M., & Spriet, L. L. (2018). Exercise metabolism: fuels for the fire. *Cold Spring Harbor perspectives in medicine, 8*(8), a029744. https://doi.org/10.1101/cshperspect.a029744

38. Alghannam, A. F., Gonzalez, J. T., & Betts, J. A. (2018). Restoration of muscle glycogen and functional capacity: role of post-exercise carbohydrate and protein co-ingestion. *Nutrients, 10*(2), 253. https://doi.org/10.3390/nu10020253

39. Burke, L. M., van Loon, L. J. C., & Hawley, J. A. (2017). Postexercise muscle glycogen resynthesis in humans. *J appl physiol (1985), 122*(5), 1055–1067. doi:10.1152/japplphysiol.00860.2016

40. Sá, M. A., Neto, G. R., Costa, P. B., Gomes, T. M., Bentes, C. M., Brown, A. F., & Novaes, J. S. (2015). Acute effects of different stretching techniques on the number of repetitions in a single lower body resistance training session. *Journal of human kinetics, 45*, 177–185. https://doi.org/10.1515/hukin-2015-0018

41. Xie, Y., Feng, B., Chen, K., Andersen, L. L., Page, P., & Wang, Y. (2018). The efficacy of dynamic contract-relax stretching on delayed-onset muscle soreness among healthy individuals: a randomized clinical trial. *Clinical journal of sport medicine: official journal of the Canadian Academy of Sport Medicine, 28*(1), 28–36. https://doi.org/10.1097/JSM.0000000000000442

42. Contrò, V., Mancuso, E. P., & Proia, P. (2016). Delayed onset muscle soreness (DOMS) management: present state of the art. *TRENDS in Sport Sciences, 3*(23), 121–127. https://core.ac.uk/download/pdf/53306674.pdf

43. Tsatsouline, P. (2001). Relax into stretch: instant flexibility through mastering muscle tension. Dragon Door Publication, 39–44.

44. Herbert, R. D., de Noronha, M., & Kamper, S. J. (2011). Stretching to prevent or reduce muscle soreness after exercise. *The Cochrane database of systematic reviews*, (7), CD004577. https://doi.org/10.1002/14651858.CD004577.pub3

45. Behm, D. G., Blazevich, A. J., Kay, A. D., & McHugh, M. (2016). Acute effects of muscle stretching on physical performance, range of motion, and injury incidence in healthy active individuals: a systematic review. *Applied physiology, nutrition, and metabolism = Physiologie appliquee, nutrition et metabolisme, 41*(1), 1–11. https://doi.org/10.1139/apnm-2015-0235

46. Page, P. (2012). Current concepts in muscle stretching for exercise and rehabilitation. *International journal of sports physical therapy, 7*(1), 109–119.

47. Hindle, K. B., Whitcomb, T. J., Briggs, W. O., & Hong, J. (2012). Proprioceptive neuromuscular facilitation (PNF): its mechanisms and effects on range of motion and muscular function. *Journal of human kinetics, 31*, 105–113. https://doi.org/10.2478/v10078-012-0011-y

48. Opplert, J., & Babault, N. (2019). Acute effects of dynamic stretching on mechanical properties result from both muscle-tendon stretching and muscle warm-up. *Journal of sports science & medicine, 18*(2), 351–358.

49. Harvey, L. A., Katalinic, O. M., Herbert, R. D., Moseley, A. M., Lannin, N. A., & Schurr, K. (2017). Stretch for the treatment and prevention of contracture: an abridged republication of a Cochrane Systematic Review. *Journal of physiotherapy, 63*(2), 67–75. https://doi.org/10.1016/j.jphys.2017.02.014

50. Burgess, K. E., Graham-Smith, P., & Pearson, S. J. (2009). Effect of acute tensile loading on gender-specific tendon structural and mechanical properties. *Journal of orthopaedic research: official publication of the Orthopaedic Research Society, 27*(4), 510–516. https://doi.org/10.1002/jor.20768

51. Thomas, E., Bianco, A., Paoli, A., & Palma, A. (2018). The relation between stretching typology and stretching duration: the effects on range of Motion. *International journal of sports medicine, 39*(4), 243–254. https://doi.org/10.1055/s-0044-101146

52. Alizadeh Ebadi, L., & Çetin, E. (2018). Duration dependent effect of static stretching on quadriceps and hamstring muscle force. *Sports, 6*(1), 24. https://doi.org/10.3390/sports6010024

53. Scott, E. E., Hamilton, D. F., Wallace, R. J., Muir, A. Y., & Simpson, A. H. (2016). Increased risk of muscle tears below physiological temperature ranges. *Bone & joint research, 5*(2), 61–65. https://doi.org/10.1302/2046-3758.52.2000484

54. Henry, F. M. (1958). Specificity vs generality in learning motor skills. *Proceedings, College Physical Education Association*, 61, 126–128.

55. Swift, D. L., Johannsen, N. M., Tudor-Locke, C., Earnest, C. P., Johnson, W. D., Blair, S. N., Sénéchal, M., & Church, T. S. (2012). Exercise training and habitual physical activity: a randomized controlled trial. *American journal of preventive medicine, 43*(6), 629–635. https://doi.org/10.1016/j.amepre.2012.08.024

56. La Scala Teixeira, C. V., Motoyama, Y., de Azevedo, P., Evangelista, A. L., Steele, J., & Bocalini, D. S. (2018). Effect of resistance training set volume on upper body muscle hypertrophy: are more sets really better than less?. *Clinical physiology and functional imaging, 38*(5), 727–732. https://doi.org/10.1111/cpf.12476

57. da Silva Vasconcelos, E., & Salla, R. F. (2018). Resistance exercise, muscle damage and inflammatory response 'what doesn't kill you makes you stronger. *MOJ sports med, 2*(2). https://www.researchgate.net/publication/323832916

58. Calle, M. C., & Fernandez, M. L. (2010). Effects of resistance training on the inflammatory response. *Nutrition research and practice, 4*(4), 259–269. https://doi.org/10.4162/nrp.2010.4.4.259

59. Enoka, R. M. (1996). Eccentric contractions require unique activation strategies by the nervous system. *Journal of applied physiology, 81*(6), 2339–2346. https://doi.org/10.1152/jappl.1996.81.6.2339

60. Vierck, J., O'Reilly, B., Hossner, K., Antonio, J., Byrne, K., Bucci, L., & Dodson, M. (2000). Satellite cell regulation following myotrauma caused by resistance exercise. *Cell biology international, 24*(5), 263–272. https://doi.org/10.1006/cbir.2000.0499

61. Damas, F., Libardi, C. A., & Ugrinowitsch, C. (2018). The development of skeletal muscle hypertrophy through resistance training: the role of muscle damage and muscle protein synthesis. *European journal of applied physiology, 118*(3), 485–500. https://doi.org/10.1007/s00421-017-3792-9

62. Nosaka, K., Lavender, A., Newton, M., & Sacco, P. (2003). Muscle damage in resistance training: is muscle damage necessary for strength gain and muscle hyper-trophy? *International journal of sports health and science, 1*(1), 1–8. https://www.jstage.jst.go.jp/article/ijshs/1/1/1_1_1/_pdf

63. Baechle, T. R., & Earle, R. W. (2008). *Essentials of strength training and conditioning* (3rd ed.). Champaign, IL: Human kinetics National Strength and Conditioning Association. https://www.worldcat.org/title/essentials-of-strength-training-and-conditioning/oclc/190867428

64. Selye, H. (1950). *The physiology and pathology of exposure to stress, a treatise based on the concepts of the general-adaptation syndrome and the diseases of adaptation.* Montreal: ACTA, Inc., Medical Publishers.

65. Delorme, T. L., West, F. E., & Shriber, W. J. (1950). Influence of progressive resistance exercises on knee function following femoral fractures. *The Journal of bone and joint surgery, American volume, 32A*(4), 910–924.

66. *Mosby's Medical Dictionary* (9th ed.). (2009). St. Louis, MO: Elsevier.

67. Knight, K. L. (1990). Quadriceps strengthening with the DAPRE technique: Case studies with neurological implications. *The Journal of orthopaedic and sports physical therapy, 12*(2), 66–71. https://doi.org/10.2519/jospt.1990.12.2.66

68. Ardali, G. (2014). A daily adjustable progressive resistance exercise protocol and functional training to increase quadriceps muscle strength and functional performance in an elderly homebound patient following a total knee arthroplasty. *Physiotherapy theory and practice, 30*(4), 287–297. https://doi.org/10.3109/09593985.2013.868064

69. Nygaard Falch, H., Guldteig Rædergård, H., & van den Tillaar, R. (2019). Effect of different physical training forms on change of direction ability: a systematic review and meta-analysis. *Sports medicine – open, 5*(1), 53. https://doi.org/10.1186/s40798-019-0223-y

70. Larsen, M. N., Nielsen, C. M., Helge, E. W., Madsen, M., Manniche, V., Hansen, L., Hansen, P. R., Bangsbo, J., & Krustrup, P. (2018). Positive effects on bone mineralisation and muscular fitness after 10 months of intense school-based physical training for children aged 8–10 years: the FIT FIRST randomised controlled trial. *British journal of sports medicine, 52*(4), 254–260. https://doi.org/10.1136/bjsports-2016-096219

71. Attwood, M. J., Roberts, S. P., Trewartha, G., England, M. E., & Stokes, K. A. (2018). Efficacy of a movement control injury prevention programme in adult men's community rugby union: a cluster randomised controlled trial. *British journal of sports medicine, 52*(6), 368–374. https://doi.org/10.1136/bjsports-2017-098005

72. Kibler, W. B., Press, J., & Sciascia, A. (2006). The role of core stability in athletic function. *Sports medicine, 36*(3), 189–198. https://doi.org/10.2165/00007256-200636030-00001

73. Hodges, P. W., Eriksson, A. E., Shirley, D., & Gandevia, S. C. (2005). Intra-abdominal pressure increases stiffness of the lumbar spine. *Journal of biomechanics, 38*(9), 1873–1880. https://doi.org/10.1016/j.jbiomech.2004.08.016

74. Beneka, A. G., Malliou, P. K., Missailidou, V., Chatzinikolaou, A., Fatouros, I., Gourgoulis, V., & Georgiadis, E. (2013). Muscle performance following an acute bout of plyometric training combined with low or high intensity weight exercise. *Journal of sports sciences, 31*(3), 335–343. https://doi.org/10.1080/02640414.2012.733820

75. Tuthill, J. C., & Azim, E. (2018). Proprioception. *Current biology, 28*(5), R194–R203. https://doi.org/10.1016/j.cub.2018.01.064

76. Costill, D. L., Maglischo, E. W., Richardson, A. B. (1992). *Handbook of sports medicine and science: Swimming.* Oxford: Blackwell Scientific Publications.

77. Coyle, E. F., Coggan, A. R., Hemmert, M. K., & Ivy, J. L. (1986). Muscle glycogen utilization during prolonged strenuous exercise when fed carbohydrate. *Journal of applied physiology, 61*(1), 165–172. https://doi.org/10.1152/jappl.1986.61.1.165

78. Devlin, J. T., Barlow, J., & Horton, E. S. (1989). Whole body and regional fuel metabolism during early postexercise recovery. *The American journal of physiology, 256*(1 pt 1), E167–E172. https://doi.org/10.1152/ajpendo.1989.256.1.E167

79. Fallowfield, J. L., Williams, C., & Singh, R. (1995). The influence of ingesting a carbohydrate-electrolyte beverage during 4 hours of recovery on subsequent endurance capacity. *International journal of sport nutrition, 5*(4), 285–299. https://doi.org/10.1123/ijsn.5.4.285

80. Ivy, J. L., Katz, A. L., Cutler, C. L., Sherman, W. M., & Coyle, E. F. (1988). Muscle glycogen synthesis after exercise: effect of time of carbohydrate ingestion. *Journal of applied physiology, 64*(4), 1480–1485. https://doi.org/10.1152/jappl.1988.64.4.1480

81. Jensen, J., Rustad, P. I., Kolnes, A. J., & Lai, Y. C. (2011). The role of skeletal muscle glycogen breakdown for regulation of insulin sensitivity by exercise. *Frontiers in physiology, 2,* 112. https://doi.org/10.3389/fphys.2011.00112

82. Bergström, J., Hermansen, L., Hultman, E., & Saltin, B. (1967). Diet, muscle glycogen and physical performance. *Acta physiologica Scandinavica, 71*(2), 140–150. https://doi.org/10.1111/j.1748-1716.1967.tb03720.x

83. Costill, D. L., Sherman, W. M., Fink, W. J., Maresh, C., Witten, M., & Miller, J. M. (1981). The role of dietary carbohydrates in muscle glycogen resynthesis after strenuous running. *The American journal of clinical nutrition, 34*(9), 1831–1836. https://doi.org/10.1093/ajcn/34.9.1831

84. Piehl, K. (1974). Glycogen storage and depletion in human skeletal muscle fibres. *Acta physiologica Scandinavica. Supplementum, 402,* 1–32.

85. Maehlum, S., Høstmark, A. T., & Hermansen, L. (1977). Synthesis of muscle glycogen during recovery after prolonged severe exercise in diabetic and non-diabetic subjects. *Scandinavian journal of clinical and laboratory investigation, 37*(4), 309–316. https://doi.org/10.3109/00365517709092634

86. Maughan, R. J., Owen, J. H., Shirreffs, S. M., & Leiper, J. B. (1994). Post-exercise rehydration in man: effects of electrolyte addition to ingested fluids. *European journal of applied physiology and occupational physiology, 69*(3), 209–215. https://doi.org/10.1007/BF01094790

87. Williams, M., Raven, P. B., Fogt, D. L., & Ivy, J. L. (2003). Effects of recovery beverages on glycogen restoration and endurance exercise performance. *Journal of strength and conditioning research, 17*(1), 12–19. https://doi.org/10.1519/1533–4287(2003)0172.0.co;2

88. Wasserman, D. H. (2009). Four grams of glucose. *American journal of physiology. Endocrinology and metabolism, 296*(1), E11–E21. https://doi.org/10.1152/ajpendo.90563.2008

89. Doyle, D. A., Morais Cabral, J., Pfuetzner, R. A., Kuo, A., Gulbis, J. M., Cohen, S. L., Chait, B. T., & MacKinnon, R. (1998). The structure of the potassium channel: molecular basis of K+ conduction and selectivity. *Science, 280*(5360), 69–77. https://doi.org/10.1126/science.280.5360.69

90. Sleiman, S. F., Henry, J., Al-Haddad, R., El Hayek, L., Abou Haidar, E., Stringer, T., Ulja, D., Karuppagounder, S. S., Holson, E. B., Ratan, R. R., Ninan, I., & Chao, M. V. (2016). Exercise promotes the expression of brain derived neurotrophic factor (BDNF) through the action of the ketone body β-hydroxybutyrate. *eLife, 5,* e15092. https://doi.org/10.7554/eLife.15092

91. Jentjens, R. L., Cale, C., Gutch, C., & Jeukendrup, A. E. (2003). Effects of pre-exercise ingestion of differing amounts of carbohydrate on subsequent metabolism and cycling performance. *European journal of applied physiology, 88*(4–5), 444–452. https://doi.org/10.1007/s00421-002-0727-9

92. Robergs, R. A. (1991). Nutrition and exercise determinants of postexercise glycogen synthesis. *International journal of sport nutrition, 1*(4), 307–337. https://doi.org/10.1123/ijsn.1.4.307

93. Ivy, J. L., Goforth, H. W., Jr., Damon, B. M., McCauley, T. R., Parsons, E. C., & Price, T. B. (2002). Early postexercise muscle glycogen recovery is enhanced with a carbohydrate-protein supplement. *Journal of applied physiology, 93*(4), 1337–1344. https://doi.org/10.1152/japplphysiol.00394.2002

94. Zawadzki, K. M., Yaspelkis, B. B. III, & Ivy, J. L. (1992). Carbohydrate-protein complex increases the rate of muscle glycogen storage after exercise. *Journal of applied physiology, 72*(5), 1854–1859. https://doi.org/10.1152/jappl.1992.72.5.1854

95. Costill, D. L., Flynn, M. G., Kirwan, J. P., Houmard, J. A., Mitchell, J. B., Thomas, R., & Park, S. H. (1988). Effects of repeated days of intensified training on muscle glycogen and swimming performance. *Medicine and science in sports and exercise, 20*(3), 249–254. https://doi.org/10.1249/00005768-198806000-00006

96. Devlin, J. T., Barlow, J., & Horton, E. S. (1989). Whole body and regional fuel metabolism during early postexercise recovery. *The American journal of physiology, 256*(1 pt 1), E167–E172. https://doi.org/10.1152/ajpendo.1989.256.1.E167

97. Ploug, T., Galbo, H., Vinten, J., Jørgensen, M., & Richter, E. A. (1987). Kinetics of glucose transport in rat muscle: effects of insulin and contractions. *The American journal of physiology, 253*(1 pt 1), E12–E20. https://doi.org/10.1152/ajpendo.1987.253.1.E12

98. Coyle, E. F., Coggan, A. R., Hemmert, M. K., & Ivy, J. L. (1986). Muscle glycogen utilization during prolonged strenuous exercise when fed carbohydrate. *Journal of applied physiology, 61*(1), 165–172. https://doi.org/10.1152/jappl.1986.61.1.165

99. Rockwell, M. S., Rankin, J. W., & Dixon, H. (2003). Effects of muscle glycogen on performance of repeated sprints and mechanisms of fatigue. *International journal of sport nutrition and exercise metabolism, 13*(1), 1–14. https://doi.org/10.1123/ijsnem.13.1.1

100. Katayama, K., Goto, K., Ishida, K., & Ogita, F. (2010). Substrate utilization during exercise and recovery at moderate altitude. *Metabolism: clinical and experimental, 59*(7), 959–966. https://doi.org/10.1016/j.metabol.2009.10.017

101. Nielsen, J., Holmberg, H. C., Schrøder, H. D., Saltin, B., & Ortenblad, N. (2011). Human skeletal muscle glycogen utilization in exhaustive exercise: role of subcellular localization and fibre type. *The Journal of physiology, 589*(pt 11), 2871–2885. https://doi.org/10.1113/jphysiol.2010.204487

102. Ørtenblad, N., Westerblad, H., & Nielsen, J. (2013). Muscle glycogen stores and fatigue. *The Journal of physiology, 591*(18), 4405–4413. https://doi.org/10.1113/jphysiol.2013.251629

103. Karp, J. R., Johnston, J. D., Tecklenburg, S., Mickleborough, T. D., Fly, A. D., & Stager, J. M. (2006). Chocolate milk as a post-exercise recovery aid. *International journal of sport nutrition and exercise metabolism, 16*(1), 78–91. https://doi.org/10.1123/ijsnem.16.1.78

104. Baldwin, K. M., Winder, W. W., & Holloszy, J. O. (1975). Adaptation of actomyosin ATPase in different types of muscle to endurance exercise. *The American journal of physiology, 229*(2), 422–426. https://doi.org/10.1152/ajplegacy.1975.229.2.422

7

PROFESSIONAL, ACADEMIC AND RESEARCH SKILLS

Konstantinos Papadopoulos

Academic Writing, Do's and Don'ts

It is really hard to give a formal definition to academic writing. Academic writing refers to a particular style of expression that scholars use to define the boundaries of their disciplines and their areas of expertise. Each academic discipline has its own specialist vocabulary which you will be expected to learn and use in your own writing. Academic writing is formal and follows some standard conventions. Characteristics of academic writing include a formal tone, use of the third-person rather than first-person perspective, and a clear focus on the problem that is investigated. Academic writing can allow you to present your argument and analysis accurately and concisely. In Table 7.1 you can find some do's and don'ts that hopefully will help you with your academic assignments [1].

What Referencing Is and How to Avoid Plagiarism

Plagiarism involves deliberately or inadvertently presenting someone else's ideas as your own. Most universities treat plagiarism very seriously. Plagiarism usually results in disciplinary action. One of the key things in order to avoid plagiarism, is referencing. Every time you are using someone's ideas, theories, data or any other material, you must make sure that you acknowledge the source by citing it in the main body and adding the full reference in the reference list. The reference list should be in the referencing style that your institution is required. There are several different referencing styles used across different institutions with the most common (in allied-health sciences) being the Harvard referencing style.

Additionally, when writing academic papers, you will be asked to not 'copy and paste' your sources (unless it is important to quote exactly what they said) but to use your own words. Expressing another person's ideas in your own words is called paraphrasing and it is a very important skill when it comes to academic writing. An easy way to paraphrase effectively is by reading a passage and then making notes. This should help you use your own words.

TABLE 7.1 Do's and Don'ts in academic writing

Do's	Don'ts
Aim for precision. Don't use unnecessary words or waffle. Get straight to the point. Make every word count.	Do not use overly elaborate language as it will make your writing seem pretentious.
Avoid over-long sentences and aim for a mixture of long and short sentences for variation and rhythm.	Do not use contractions (it's, doesn't, hasn't).
Avoid repeating the same words.	Do not use colloquial expressions such as 'As I was saying' or 'As a matter of fact'.
Use technical language and words specific to your discipline.	Do not use categorical statements. Instead phrase statements using verbs such as 'might' or 'may' or adverbs such as 'perhaps' or 'possibly'.
Avoid conversational terms (totally) and choose more appropriate words (significantly).	Do not use abbreviations (unless the abbreviation has previously been explained).
Avoid vague terms (nice, popular)	Do not use first person sentences (I, we).
Use impersonal sentences (Consideration has been given ...).	Do not forget to reference and add a reference list at the end of your academic assignment.
Make sure your work is well presented, in the correct word font and size, it has been proofread and it is within the word limit.	Do not get rushed but make sure you spend the expected amount of time for the completion of your work.

Critiquing Research and Developing Critical Thinking and Analytical Skills

Most of you have been (or will be) in a position that required you to deal with a new (non-crucial) situation at work. What did you do? Did you ask your peers, look it up on the web or try to find your answer in a peer-reviewed journal? Research has shown that the most common response to this would be a quick question or phone call to one of your peers [2]. Although looking things up on the web or asking our peers seems to be the easiest way to tackle uncertain situations, this information might not be the most accurate, or based on research. Evidence that comes after critical peer-review (evidence-based) is the safest option and what should inform our practice. It is also the only acceptable source when it comes to academic writing. However, although a research study is published in a peer-reviewed journal, this does not mean it is perfect as the researcher often has to balance conflicting and complex demands. We, therefore, need to be critical readers of such evidence. The function of a critique is not to describe a study but to appraise its worth and merits. As a critical reader you will need to be able to identify and comment on the strength and weaknesses. You will need to justify your criticisms, offer a rationale of how a limitation affected the quality of the study and suggest an alternate approach to eliminate the problem. Avoid vague generalisations and be as objective as possible.

Although reading scientific papers and critiquing them appears to be time-consuming, adopting the following four-step approach of critical appraisal might help you get the information you need easier.

1. Quick skim (familiarise yourself)
2. Skilled reading to understand different parts of study (question, aims, sample, method of data collection, ethical issues, method of analysis, main results/findings, interpretation and conclusions)

3. Each part of study is broken down and appraised in terms of its merit
4. All parts are reconstituted. Consider overall impact of study (Adopted and modified from LoBiondo-Wood and Haber) [3]

Self-Reflection as Part of Professional Skills

Another part of professional and critical skills is self-reflection which has emerged as a reoccurring theme in many allied-health professions in the last several decades. Specifically, reflective practices have been used in nursing, occupational therapy and speech language pathology. Sport practitioners also use reflection in order to improve patient care, support clinical supervision, improve collaboration and advance clinical reasoning. Self-reflection can give you a sense of discomfort [4] so it is no wonder many people put it off and may even try to get by without it. Reflecting on your actions is something that requires conscious effort after the event but eventually it will become an automatic thought process even when you're in the middle of experiencing the event. Literature reports different models of reflection. Below you will find the two most common reflective models used by sport practitioners.

Gibbs Reflective Cycle [5] encourages people to think systematically about the experiences they had during a specific situation, event or activity. Using a circle, reflection on those experiences can be structured in phases. This often makes people think about an experience, activity or event in more detail, making them aware of their own actions and better able to adjust and change their behaviour. By looking at both negative and positive impacts of the event, people can learn from it.

The cycle starts with description and then continues clockwise to feelings, evaluation, analysis, conclusion and action plan, to finally return to description (Figure 7.1); however, the model has been criticised for being a superficial reflection with no referral to critical thinking/analysis/assumptions or viewing it from a different perspective [6].

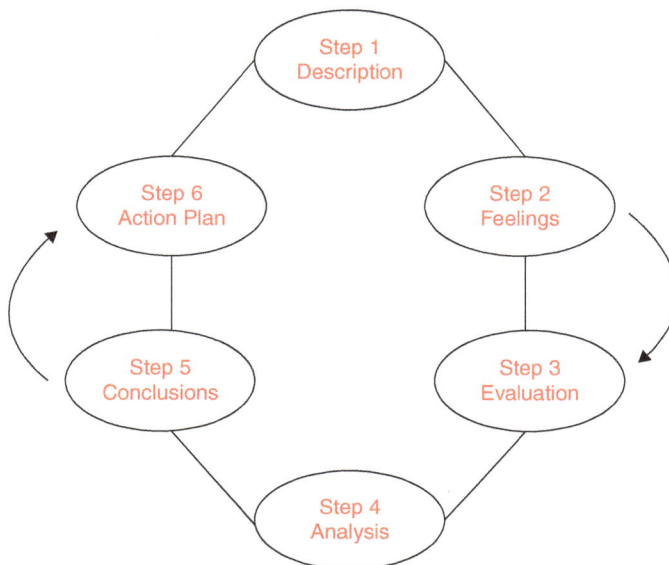

FIGURE 7.1 Gibbs Reflective Cycle (adopted from Gibbs, 1998) [5].

The second reflective model comes from Rolfe et al. [7]. Their reflective model is based upon three simple questions: What? So what? Now what? but repeats these questions at three levels, with increasingly deeper reflection at each level. The levels are descriptive, theoretical and action-orientated. Working through the same questions at different levels can be used to develop from novice to expert; however, it may be too complicated for a beginner who is new to reflection.

Communicating Academic Ideas to Peers and Other Professionals

Academic papers should be considered as forms of communications between scholars. There has always been a need to communicate academic ideas; it pools knowledge on knowledge to afford us a background to find the answers that we previously did not manage to find [8]. The most common forms for scientific communications are journal articles, proposals, theses, abstracts, speeches, or lectures, poster presentations, but also books, review papers and group communications. Regardless of the form of communication, the most important thing that scientists think of first is their audience. Understanding your audience and your position relative to the audience are crucial issues to the success of any communication [8]. The language, the content, the level of detail, the layout and the mode of delivery depend on how familiar your audience is with your topic. Therefore, the first thing to ask when trying to communicate ideas is: who is your target audience? Is it your peers who are also experts in the field? Is it peers with a different research focus or colleagues from other professions?

Additionally, each form of communication is used for a different purpose. For example, a thesis is a long essay embodying results of original research and especially substantiating a specific view written by a candidate for a university degree. On the other hand, a research proposal aims to convince the reader of the value of your project and your competence and is likely to lead to a funding opportunity. The most common way to communicate academic ideas is by publishing research papers in scientific journals. Before this happens, the research is reviewed by peers who are experts in the field and will determine whether the research evidence should be published or not. All research papers do not follow the same principles. Depending on the research question that needs to be answered researchers have to choose from different research methodologies.

Research Methodologies and Designs

A research hypothesis is a specific, clear and testable proposition or predictive statement about the possible outcome of a scientific research study based on a particular property of a population, such as presumed differences between groups on a particular variable or relationships between variables. Specifying the research hypotheses is one of the most important steps in planning a scientific quantitative research study. Usually, researchers report the null hypothesis which is a general statement or default position that there is no relationship between two measured phenomena or no association among groups. The study then aims to identify whether the hypothesis needs to be accepted or rejected [9].

The researcher needs to identify the right research methodology which will be able assessment of the research hypothesis. There are two main research methodologies: **quantitative** and **qualitative**. Quantitative research methods focus on collecting and analysing data that is structured and can be represented numerically. One of the central goals is to build accurate and reliable measurements that allow for statistical analysis [10]. Qualitative research is a method in which the researcher collects textual material derived from speech or observation and attempts to understand the phenomena of interest in terms of the meanings people bring to them [11]. Qualitative research focuses on experience, feelings, opinion, knowledge and input. Mixed methods research capitalises on the strengths of both qualitative and quantitative methodology by combining both components in a single research study to increase breadth and depth of understanding [12].

What Is Research Design?

A research design is a specific plan or protocol for conducting the study, which allows the investigator to translate the conceptual hypothesis into an operational one [13].

The main **qualitative** research designs in sports and health sciences are ethnography, grounded theory and phenomenology.

Ethnography

This research design seeks to describe and interpret social groups from the viewpoint of an insider. It has roots in anthropology and is used to study all manner of social relationships and realities, e.g. describing the lives of people living with disability. Ethnography focuses on three activities: 1) what the people in the group are doing, 2) the things that have meaning to the group and what those things are, 3) what the people in the group say. To collect these data the ethnographer uses observation techniques and engages with the group in a number of different ways using things that have a meaning to the group such as pictures, symbols and images. The researcher becomes both an observer and a participant [14].

Grounded Theory

This research design is used to analyse social processes that occur within human interactions. It aims to generate new or expand upon existing ideas, theories about a human activity and is used to generate theories about practice from different areas of healthcare, e.g. gaining insights into how people learn to adapt to life after a sports injury. Grounded theory is the most systematic and the most popular. It uses theory-building strategies and the main collection methods are unstructured or semi-structured interviews of a homogeneous sample [15].

Phenomenology

Phenomenology is the study of structures of consciousness as experienced from the first point of view. It aims to access the essence of an object or an experience as the individual experiencing it, no more and no less. Phenomenology studies the individual's lived experiences and events, e.g. the experience of AIDS care. Collection methods include flexible interviewing structures which can explore the meaning of essence of an experience [16].

The main **quantitative** research designs in sports and health sciences can be found in Figure 7.2

Editorials and Expert Opinion Reports

The lowest evidence-based research includes editorials and expert opinion reports. The purpose of such a report would be to provide an expert opinion in a field of debate, to indicate points to consider in a decision process and to compile the existing knowledge relevant for the answer to a question or the solution to a problem [17].

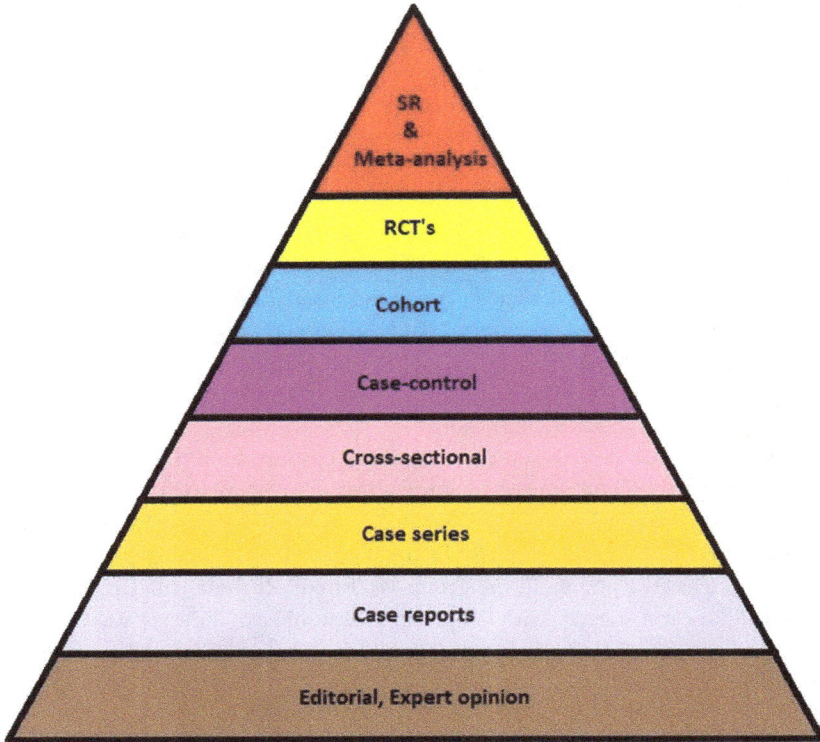

FIGURE 7.2 Research design pyramid.

Case Reports and Case Series

These are study designs which include a detailed presentation of a single case or a group of patients with the same diagnosis respectively. Cases may be identified from a single or multiple source and they are usually new or unique cases which cannot be used to study cause and effect relationships or to assess disease frequency [18].

Cross-Sectional Studies

This is an observational design that surveys exposures and disease status at a single point of time (cross-sectional of the population). This design is often used to study conditions that are relatively frequent with duration of expression (non-fatal, chronic conditions). As a result, these studies are not suitable for studying rare or highly fatal diseases or a disease with a short duration of expression. Cross-sectional designs give a general description or scope of a problem and they can be very useful in health service evaluation and planning [19].

A Case-Control Study

This is another observational study design comparing exposures in disease cases vs healthy controls from the same population. It is the most feasible design where disease outcomes are rare and where the exposure data can be collected retrospectively. This design allows the examination of multiple exposures; they are suitable for rare diseases with long latency and can be conducted when randomised studies are unethical [9].

A Cohort Study

This type of study is considered the highest amongst the observational study designs. This design compares individuals with a known risk factor or exposure with others without the risk factor or exposure. Cohort studies are looking for a difference in the risk of a disease over time. Data are usually collected prospectively and multiple outcomes can be studied. Although these studies can establish population-based incidence and can estimate relative risks accurately [20], they are usually lengthy and expensive, may require long samples and are not suitable for rare diseases.

A Randomised Controlled Trial (RCT)

RCTs are experimental (not observational) designs where a treatment or an exposure occurs in a 'controlled' environment. They consist of the 'gold standard' of research designs when it comes to primary collected data. The design generally involves random assignment of subjects to treatment and comparison groups. It provides most convincing evidence of relationship between exposure and effect; however, if the exposure can be harmful then this design cannot be used due to ethical reasons [21].

Systematic Reviews (SR)

Systematic reviews are those research designs which aim to summarise the results of available carefully designed healthcare studies (controlled trials) and provide a high level of evidence on the effectiveness of healthcare interventions. Systematic reviews differ from traditional narrative reviews which are mainly descriptive. Systematic reviews, as the name implies, typically involve a detailed and comprehensive plan and search strategy derived a priori, with the goal of reducing bias by identifying, appraising and synthesising all relevant studies on a particular topic [22]. Often, systematic reviews include a meta-analysis component which involves using statistical techniques to synthesise the data from several studies into a single quantitative estimate or summary effect size [23].

Statistics as Part of a Research Project

All science is based on precise and consistent measurement. Whether or not you consider yourself to be an exercise therapist or a physical education lecturer, or a strength and conditioning coach, there is a lot to gain by learning proper measurement techniques. A *measurement* is the process of comparing value to a standard. When a lecturer tests students in the isokinetic dynamometer the process of measurement is being applied. The result of this process will give the lecturer a bit of information about how strong each student is. This information is called *data*. Different bits of data cannot always give the information we need; therefore, data are usually organised by a process called **statistics**.

In sport and health sciences, the use of statistical tests to analyse data and determine whether the null hypothesis needs to be rejected or not is probably the most common way. Some statistical tests can be performed by hand, but most of them would require a significant amount of time and statistical knowledge (especially with large data sets). In addition, even with the simpler tests, it is not difficult to select a wrong option and obtain inappropriate results. For that reason, researchers, most of the time, use a statistical software for their data analysis. This software is very important to researchers but also to students who have to conduct a research project as part of their dissertation module. The statistical package will enable them to understand and use the most important part of the output. Additionally, students need to be able to present their results in their dissertation, with appropriate tables and charts. One of the most common statistical packages used in sport and healthcare sciences is the SPSS (Statistical Package for the Social Sciences). This package gives you a variety of options and statistical analyses. It includes several statistical tests which can be used to describe data and answer any research hypotheses.

Key Word Definitions

The **mean** is the statistical name for the arithmetic average. It is the most commonly used measure of central tendency. Its calculation considers both the number of scores and their values. The mean gives weight to each score according to its relative distance from other scores in the data set. It is calculated by summing all scores and dividing the sum by the number of scores (N). Summing scores are presented by the symbol Σ, which is the uppercase figure for the Greek character sigma. Therefore, if a variable is labelled X, then ΣX should be the read 'the sum of X'. To denote the mean of a variable, we place a line over the symbol for the variable $(\bar{X})$, *often read as 'X-bar'. Then, the formula should be:*

$$\bar{X} = \Sigma X/N$$

The **mode** is the score that occurs most frequently. It can be found if we scan the list of all our scores and identify the one that is the most frequent. No formula can calculate it. Knowing the mode, we can easily estimate the centre of the group and whether the distribution is normal or nearly normal. However, it is important to note that the mode might disregard the extreme scores and it cannot be used for further calculations.

The **median** is the middle score. It divides the data set in half; therefore, it is associated with the 50th percentile. The median can easily show us which scores represents the majority of the other values. As you can see below, in a rank order distribution, the median is the middle score when N is odd, whilst when N is even the median falls between two scores.

A	B
9	19
8	18
Median→ 6 ←Median	
4	17
1	16

The median does not consider the size of scores, but only how many there are. It is based only on the number of scores and their rank order. For that reason, the median should be used on ordinal data and on data that are highly skewed.

Standard Deviation (SD) is the most common method of measuring the variability, or dispersion, of a data set. It considers the deviation (distance) from the mean value. SD is the square root of the average of the squared deviation from the mean. When the SD is small the data set is more compact. When it is large, there is more diversity. Normally, there are usually five or six SDs within the range of data set considering that the distribution is normal. If there are more, then the researchers should check the calculations for errors.

A normal distribution (Figure 7.3) curve is bilaterally symmetrical and is shaped like a bell. However, not all symmetrical curves are normally distributed. A normal distribution is when most subjects score in the middle range. The two ends, or tails, of the curve are symmetrical and they represent the scores at the low and high extremes of the scale.

In a skewed curve, the median and mean are not the same, as is the case with a bell curve. In a positively skewed curve, the large number of smaller values makes the median smaller than the mean, which is affected by the high values in the tail of the distribution. On the opposite side, a negatively skewed distribution has a greater number of higher values, with the tail heading off to the left. In this type of distribution, the median is greater than the mean (Figure 7.3).

What type of statistical test to use for the analysis of our research also depends on the distribution of the data. Parametric and nonparametric are two broad classifications of statistical procedures. Parametric tests are based on assumptions about the distribution of the underlying population from which the sample was taken. The most common parametric assumption is that data are approximately normally distributed. The parametric assumption of normality is particularly worrisome for small sample sizes (n < 30). Nonparametric tests are often a good option for these data. Nonparametric tests do not rely on any distribution. They can thus be applied even if parametric conditions of validity are not met. If the data deviate strongly from the assumptions of a parametric procedure, using the parametric procedure could lead to incorrect conclusions. The tests to determine if the data are parametric or nonparametric are statistical tests such as Kolmogorov-Smirnov and Shapiro-Wilk. Informally, normal distribution can be also assessed via visual methods (P-P, Q-Q plots) or by comparing SD and means. If the assumptions of the parametric procedure are not valid, use an analogous nonparametric procedure instead [24].

Parametric tests are used only where a normal distribution is assumed. The most widely used tests are the t-tests; independent samples t-test; when two different groups are being compared at a particular time and paired (or dependent) t-tests; when one group or entity is measured twice, resulting in pairs of observations. The one-way analysis of variance (ANOVA) is used to determine whether there are any statistically significant differences between the means of three or more independent (unrelated) groups. Repeated measures ANOVA is the equivalent of the one-way ANOVA, but for related, not independent groups, and is the extension of the paired (dependent)

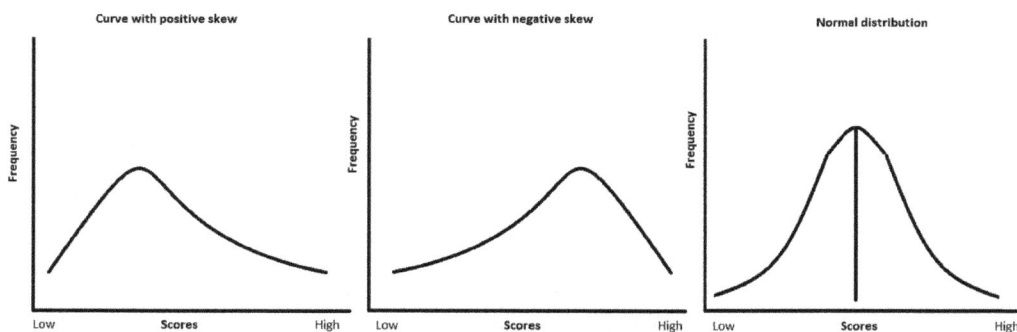

FIGURE 7.3   Positive, negative and normal distribution.

t-test. The two-way ANOVA compares the mean differences between groups that have been split on two independent variables (called factors). If the factors are three then it is named three-way ANOVA Pearson correlation coefficient is a measure of the strength of a linear association between two variables and is denoted by r. Finally, Linear regression is the next step up after Pearson correlation. It is used when we want to predict the value of a variable based on the value of another variable [25].

Nonparametric tests are used when continuous data are not normally distributed or when dealing with discrete variables. Most widely used are chi-squared, Fisher's exact tests, Wilcoxon's matched pairs, Mann–Whitney U-tests, Kruskal–Wallis tests and Spearman rank correlation [26].

The advantage of using a parametric test instead of a nonparametric equivalent is that the former will have more statistical power than the latter. In other words, a parametric test is more able to lead to a rejection of a null hypothesis. Most of the time, the p-value associated to a parametric test will be lower than the p-value associated to a nonparametric equivalent that is run on the same data.

Ethical and Moral Requirements of Research

More and more sport practitioners are being involved in research. Most of them conduct their first research project as part of their undergraduate (BSc) or postgraduate (MSc/PhD) programme. However, some of them even decide to work full-time as research fellows or as members in a research team [27]. Whether the sport practitioner is the principal investigator of a research project or is collecting data for another researcher, there are responsibilities regarding the ethics and governance of research on humans. This is why many of the professional bodies have developed codes of conduct that include research ethics for the guidance and regulation of their members.

Research ethics is a key process in ensuring the integrity of a research project (Department of Health, 2001). If research ethics are not considered when planning and conducting research the following could occur:

- The research participants could be physical, socially, emotionally or economically harmed
- The scientific value of the research could be compromised
- The reputation of the researcher/university/organisation could be harmed
- The researchers could be harmed

The Declaration of Helsinki

Several unethical projects were conducted in past such as the Tuskegge study (1932–1972) where American researchers purposely withheld treatment from 399 African-American people with syphilis for the sole purpose of studying the long-term effects of the disease, or the Willowbrook study (1963–1966) where children with developmental disabilities were deliberately infected with hepatitis (some were even fed faecal matter). Purpose of the study was to examine the course of the disease and to test a potential immunisation

As a response to these and many other unethical research studies, the research society decided to protect the wider community by establishing various conventions and international agreements on the ethical conduct of research involving human participants. The most well-known is probably the declaration of Helsinki which was first published in 1964 by the 18th general assembly of the World Medical Association (WMA) and was recently revised during the 64th general assembly of WMA in October, 2013.

There are three key tenets of the declaration of Helsinki:

* Studies should be of a generally acceptable scientific standard
* The study should cause no harm
* The study subjects should have given their full consent

Having these three tenets as a guide, many tried to identify key ethical principles and basic human rights that should be used as framework to appraise research designs. According to Beauchamp & Childress [28] the principles that should be followed throughout a research study are the following:

Beneficence. The underlying principle in health care and applies equally to research. It requires the researcher to maximise benefits and minimise the risk. If there is no benefit to the patient or to society the research is deemed unethical.

Non-maleficence. Harm may be physical psychological, social, economic, legal or harm to dignity. Researchers must make sure that they minimise the potential harms. Research subjects should be appropriately informed of the risk of potential harms

Fidelity. Researchers have the 'duty' to keep promises and must do as they said they will do. It is the researcher's responsibility to ensure the participant understands the risks.

Justice or fairness. The way of viewing the moral and ethical obligations of human beings. Applies particularly to recruitment of participants.

Veracity. Researchers should tell the truth and pass on information in a comprehensive and objective way. There may be a methodological reason for limited disclosure but this must be carefully justified.

Confidentiality. The protection of the confidentiality is a key element of research ethics in sport and rehabilitation sciences. Participants expect that their details will not be identifiable when the findings of the research will be published and that participating to research will not lead to a breach of confidentiality.

Respect for autonomy. This principle is usually associated with letting or enabling participants to make their own decisions about which health care intervention they will or not receive. Therefore, if the study they participate in is used a randomised methodology, participants should be happy with all the interventions they might have to receive.

Informed consent. Informed consent is a concept familiar to health and social care practitioners, particularly with reference to treatment and care [27]. Research participants should know that they are taking part in research; their written consent should be given at all times. The written consent confirms that the participant has been informed about the objectives of the study (most times by receiving a participant information sheet). The consent protects participants by assuring them that they can withdraw at any time during the study without having to give a reason.

The above principles apply to every stage of the research process and are closely linked.

How to Write a Research Proposal

The aim of a research proposal is twofold: to present and give a rationale for studying a research problem and to fully report the methodology (practical ways) in which the proposed research will be conducted. The study design and methods for conducting research are controlled by standards of the main discipline in which the research problem resides.

A research proposal should include an extensive literature covering the background and the reasoning behind the decision to conduct the research and a statement of the expected outcomes and benefits derived from the study's completion for both the profession and future research studies [29].

In particular, a research proposal should:

- Justify the chosen research project
- Describe the current state of knowledge on the research topic, considering all important relevant literature
- Formulate the hypothesis or research question
- Define the research strategy and methodology to be used to test the hypothesis or research question
- Discuss ethical considerations about the research methodology
- Define realistic, feasible, operational planning, based on the research methodology and general conditions
- Inform potential collaborating institutions and persons about the research project and enable them to identify the kind of support they can give
- Serve as an important tool for monitoring the research [30]

Common Mistakes to Avoid

One of the most common mistakes when writing a research proposal is not setting clear and well-structured statements to express objectives in a specific, measurable and achievable format [31]. Typically, writing objectives as SMART (Specific, Measurable, Attainable, Realistic and Time-bound) statements is the gold standard for goal setting, because it gives a clear direction for action planning and implementation [32]. Therefore, when attempting to set the objectives of a research proposal the questions that need to be answered are the following:

> **Specific**: Is there a clear action and expected result for the objective?
> **Measurable**: Can the objective be described with numbers for monitoring and evaluation?
> **Achievable**: Is it possible to meet the objective with the time and resources available?
> **Relevant**: Is the objective in line with the goal?
> **Time-bound**: Is there a deadline?

Other common mistakes to avoid when writing a research proposal:

- Failure to be concise; being 'all over the map' without a clear sense of purpose
- Failure to cite landmark works in the literature review
- Failure to delimit the contextual boundaries of the research [e.g. time, place, people, etc.]
- Failure to develop a coherent and persuasive argument for the proposed research
- Failure to stay focused on the research problem; going off on unrelated tangents
- Sloppy or imprecise writing, or poor grammar
- Too much detail on minor issues, but not enough detail on major issues

What Are the Required Skills when Writing a Research Proposal?

A research proposal requires skills in thinking and designing an academic piece of work. A research proposal is a major part of any research and includes all the key elements involved in designing a completed research study. The only difference from a completed research study is that a research proposal does not report any results of the study and the analysis of those results [33].

Beginning the Proposal Process

A good place to begin is to ask yourself a series of questions:

*   What do I want to study?
*   Where am I going to conduct the research?
*   Why is the topic important?
*   How is it significant within the subject areas covered in my class?
*   What problems will it help solve?
*   How does it build upon (and hopefully go beyond) research already conducted on the topic?
*   Can I find the participants needed for this study?
*   Who else do I need to involve?
*   What are the available resources?
*   Can I get the right equipment for this research project?
*   Can I get it done in the time available?

What Are the Sections of the Research Proposal?

1. Title of the Research Project

The title of the research proposal can be considered to be one of the most important elements of the write-up. The working title should describe the content and direction of the project. Typically, the title should include three elements that are tightly related to the objectives of the study. The title should include:

*   The population under investigation
*   The intervention that is being tested
*   The outcome measures
*   The study design

2. Introduction and Literature Review

The introduction and literature review should justify the hypothesis of the proposed research. It should summarise the relevance of the topic and give an overview of the status of international research in related areas. In other words, the introduction should report what it is already known by critically appraising previous research. Both primary and secondary studies can be used in this section; however, the results of previous Systematic Reviews are highly preferred because they summarise and analyse data from a number of studies that are included in the review [34].

3. Aims, Objectives and Null Hypothesis

This section should be well-linked to the section above. The aims should cover what the goals of this research are. Usually, the introduction and literature review section reveal a research gap that needs to be bridged. The aims of the research proposal should demonstrate what the study is planned to investigate. The study can have more than one aims and should be listed in logical sequence. Aims set out what you hope to achieve at the end of the project; the objectives, on the other hand, should be specific statements that define measurable outcomes and should report the steps and tools that will be used to achieve the desired outcomes. The null hypothesis is a general statement or default position that there is no relationship between two measured phenomena or no association among groups [35]. The null hypothesis is generally assumed to be true until evidence indicates otherwise.

4. Methodology

The researcher should choose the methodology based on the research question. In other words, the researcher's selection of an appropriate research methodology is dependent on the research question itself and how best it is addressed. The methodology should be sufficiently detailed so that it could be replicated. The methodology may include quantitative and/or qualitative approaches. In this section the researcher needs to clearly describe what study design is going to be used. The methodology should always be written in the future tense [33].

5. Materials

This section includes the description of materials or subjects used for the study. Specific elements of the data collection instruments (questionnaires, surveys, interviews, observations and equipment) should be identified and their intended plan of use outlined. The rationale for their selections should be provided.

It is very important to:

- Validate the research outcomes, by allowing other researchers to reproduce or replicate the study (one of the tenets of science)
- Specify how the ethical and/or data protection requirements of engaging human or animal subjects are being safeguarded
- Allow applicability of the research findings of your study to other future researchers and/or to evidence-based clinical practice approach

Recruitment of Human Subjects

The researcher needs to make sure that the proposal includes all the information required for a safe human subject recruitment. This would normally include:

- The characteristics of the human participants and their numbers
- Clear description of the inclusion and exclusion criteria for participants
- How participants will be approached; by whom and via which communication channel (In-person, phone call, email, text, social media)
- Potential risks or harm, as well as benefits and participant rights should be provided in unequivocal layman's terms in the participant's information sheet
- Timeline of the observations and how long their participation will be
- Who will be able to access the data after its collection, how long it will be stored for and how subject identity will be protected?
- The need for the participants to give consent and making clear they know their legal right and obligations

1. Methods

This section should describe the steps based on the methodology used (quantitative and/or qualitative) to investigate the research problem and the justification for the application of specific actions, tools or techniques used. For example, how is data going to be collected? How many times will the participants have to attend? For how long? What are the human logistic and financial resources? If possible, a flow-diagram with all the necessary steps should be included. If the approach is a replicate from previous research studies, then additional citations need to be used to attribute the cited material to the rightful author [34].

2. Statistical Analysis

This section needs to clearly describe the proposed statistical analysis or the qualitative approach that will be used for the data analysis of the study. The statistical analysis depends on the study design, the number of groups involved and the number of dependent and independent variables. This is a very important part of the proposal as any failure to propose an appropriate data analysis way lead to inappropriate results and conclusions, thereby wasting precious time [36].

3. Expected Outcomes

This section should clarify what you expect your project to deliver and why it is worth pursuing. Any benefits to sport therapy/rehabilitation field form positive expected outcomes or innovative applications of knowledge needs to be highlighted.

4. Timetable

This section indicates the timeframe for each broad stage considering literature reviews, ethics, data collection, production, modelling, review analysis, testing, reporting and proposal submission.

5. References and Bibliography

A list with all the research references and bibliography should be reported at the end, using the suggested referencing formatting which should be used throughout the research proposal.

References

1. Stott, R. (2001). The essay writing process. In Stott, R., Snaith, A., & Rylance, R. (eds), *Making your case: A practical guide to essay writing*. Harlow: Pearson Education.
2. Papadopoulos, K. D., Noyes, J., Barnes, M., Jones, J. G., & Thom, J. M. (2012). How do physiotherapists assess and treat patellofemoral pain syndrome in North Wales? A mixed-method study. *International journal of therapy and rehabilitation, 19*(5), 261–272.
3. LoBiondo-Wood, G., & Haber, J. (2018). *Nursing research: Methods and critical appraisal for evidence-based practice* (7th ed.). St. Louis, MO: Elsevier.
4. Boyd, E., & Fales, A. (1983). Reflective learning: key to learning from experience. *Journal of humanistic psychology, 23*(2), 99–117.
5. Gibbs, G. (1988). *Learning by doing: A guide to teaching and learning methods*. Oxford: Oxford Further Education Unit.
6. Atkins, S., & Murphy, K. (1995). Reflective practice. *Nursing standard, 9*(45), 2–8.

7. Rolfe, G., Freshwater, D. & Jasper, M. (2001). *Critical reflection in nursing and the helping professions: A user's guide*. Basingstoke: Palgrave Macmillan.

8. Davis, M., Davis, K. J., & Dunagan, M. M. (2012). *Scientific papers and presentations*. Waltham, MA: Academic Press.

9. Lavrakas, P. J. (2011). *Encyclopedia of survey research methods*. Thousand Oaks, CA: SAGE Publications.

10. Matthews, B., Ross, L., & Askews and Holts. (2010). *Research methods: A practical guide for the social sciences*. Harlow: Pearson Education.

11. Bradley, E. H., Curry, L. A., & Devers, K. J. (2007). *Qualitative data analysis for health services research: Developing taxonomy, themes, and theory*. Oxford: Blackwell Science.

12. Johnson, R. B., Onwuegbuzie, A. J., & Turner, L. A. (2007). Toward a definition of mixed methods research. *Journal of mixed methods research, 1*(2), 112–133. doi:10.1177/1558689806298224

13. Creswell, J. W., & Creswell, J. D. (2019). *Research design: Qualitative, quantitative, and mixed methods approaches*. Thousand Oaks, CA: SAGE Publications.

14. Atkinson, P., & Hammersley, M. (2005). Ethnography and participant observation. In Denzin, N. K., & Lincoln, Y. S. (eds), *The SAGE handbook of qualitative research*. Thousand Oaks, CA: SAGE Publications.

15. Orlikowski, W. J. (1993). CASE tools as organizational change: investigating incremental and radical changes in systems development. *Management information systems quarterly, 17*(3), 309.

16. Smith, J. A. (2004). Reflecting on the development of interpretative phenomenological analysis and its contribution to qualitative research in psychology. *Qualitative research in psychology, 1*(1), 39–54.

17. Booth, W. C., Colomb, G. G., & Williams, J. M. (2003). *The craft of research*. Chicago: University of Chicago Press.

18. Boslaugh, S. (2008). *Encyclopedia of epidemiology* (vols 1–2). Thousand Oaks, CA: SAGE Publications. doi:10.4135/9781412953948

19. Vogt, W. P. (2005). *Dictionary of statistics & methodology*. Thousand Oaks, CA: SAGE Publications. doi:10.4135/9781412983907

20. Jupp, V. (2006). *The SAGE dictionary of social research methods*. London: SAGE Publications. doi:10.4135/9780857020116

21. Bickman, L., & Reich, S. (2015). Randomized controlled trials. In Donaldson, S., Christie, C., & Mark, M. (eds), *Credible and actionable evidence*. Thousand Oaks, CA: SAGE Publications. doi:10.4135/9781483385839

22. Uman, L. S. (2011). Systematic reviews and meta-analyses. *Journal of the Canadian Academy of Child and Adolescent Psychiatry = Journal de l'Academie canadienne de psychiatrie de l'enfant et de l'adolescent, 20*(1), 57–59.

23. Petticrew, M., & Roberts, H. (2012). *Systematic reviews in the social sciences: A practical guide*. Malden, MA: Blackwell.

24. Rosner, B. (2000). *Fundamentals of biostatistics*. Pacific Grove, CA: Duxbury Press.

25. Ntoumanis, N. (2003). *A step-by-step guide to SPSS for sport and exercise studies: A step-by-step guide for students*. London: Routledge.

26. Treleaven, J., & Barrett, A. J. (2009). *Hematopoietic stem cell transplantation in clinical practice*. Edinburgh: Churchill Livingstone/Elsevier.

27. Moule, P., & Hek, G. (2011). *Making sense of research: An introduction for health and social care practitioners*. Los Angeles, CA: SAGE.

28. Beauchamp, T. L., & Childress, J. F. (2019). *Principles of biomedical ethics* (7th ed.). New York: Oxford University Press.

29. Krathwohl, D. R., & Smith, N. L. (2005). *How to prepare a dissertation proposal: Suggestions for students in education and the social and behavioral sciences*. Syracuse, NY: Syracuse University Press.

30. Gross, R., Karyadi, D., Sastroamidjojo, S., & Schultink, W. (1998). Guidelines for the development of research proposals following a structured, holistic approach for a research proposal (SHARP). *Food and nutrition bulletin, 19*(3), 268–282.

31. Day, T., & Tosey, P. (2011). Beyond SMART? A new framework for goal setting. *Curriculum journal, 22*(4), 515–534.

32. CDC Division of TB Elimination (2017). Writing SMART objectives. tinyurl.com/yar6opap (accessed 19 June 2020).

33. Attard, N. (2018). WASP (Write a scientific paper): Writing an academic research proposal. *Early human development*, 123, 39–41. https://doi.org/10.1016/j.earlhumdev.2018.04.011
34. Hollins, M. C. J., & Fleming, V. (2010). A 15-step model for writing a research proposal. *British journal of midwifery, 18*(12), 791–798.
35. Stockburger, D. W. (2007). Hypothesis and hypothesis testing. In Salkind, N.J. (ed.), *Encyclopedia of measurement and statistics.* Thousand Oaks, CA: SAGE Publications.
36. Simpson, S. H. (2015). Creating a data analysis plan: what to consider when choosing statistics for a study. *The Canadian journal of hospital pharmacy, 68*(4), 311–317. https://doi.org/10.4212/cjhp.v68i4.1471

INDEX

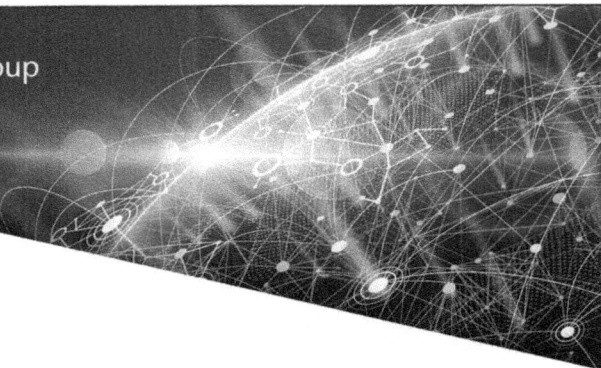

For Product Safety Concerns and Information please contact our EU
representative GPSR@taylorandfrancis.com
Taylor & Francis Verlag GmbH, Kaufingerstraße 24, 80331 München, Germany

www.ingramcontent.com/pod-product-compliance
Lightning Source LLC
Chambersburg PA
CBHW081106220326
41598CB00038B/7246

* 9 7 8 0 3 6 7 7 7 3 9 0 8 *